CARDIOLOGY RESEARCH AND CLINICAL DEVELOPMENTS

THE REDISCOVERED TRICUSPID VALVE

STRUCTURE, FUNCTION AND CLINICAL SIGNIFICANCE IN HEALTH AND DISEASE

Cardiology Research and Clinical Developments

Additional books and e-books in this series can be found on Nova's website under the Series tab.

CARDIOLOGY RESEARCH AND CLINICAL DEVELOPMENTS

THE REDISCOVERED TRICUSPID VALVE

STRUCTURE, FUNCTION AND CLINICAL SIGNIFICANCE IN HEALTH AND DISEASE

GIACOMO BIANCHI
EDITOR

nova
Medicine & Health
New York

Library of Congress Cataloging-in-Publication Data

ISBN: 978-1-53616-098-7
Library of Congress Control Number:2019947959

Published by Nova Science Publishers, Inc. † New York

CONTENTS

PREFACE

The tricuspid valve and its pathology are one of the still little known and understood aspects of cardiac physiology and pathophysiology.

In this book I have tried to gather the most significant evidence about this unknown world.

To the reader, in my mind the clinician, the cardiologist and the surgeon, I hope to give material and ideas usable in daily practice.

In the first chapter I tried to trace the development of the conception of the cardiovascular system from the galenism to Harvey's illumination, up to the first steps in understanding the physiology and pathophysiology of the tricuspid valve and the right heart.

In the second chapter, in collaboration with the anatomo-pathologist, I traced the embryological phases of the development of the valve and its morphological description, since this is where the foundations of the clinical and surgical anatomy are laid, which I also mention in the general context of the special pathology.

The third chapter, which is more clinical in nature, systematizes the epidemiology and the clinic of significant diseases of the tricuspid valve, the diagnostic approach and the recommendations on how to set up a therapeutic path.

The fourth and fifth chapters are dedicated to imaging. In particular, the fourth chapter evaluates transthoracic and transesophageal echocardiography, which are the cornerstone of the diagnosis and evaluation of tricuspid valve disease. The fifth chapter focuses on third level imaging techniques such as Magnetic Resonance Imaging and CT scanning; these techniques allow to merge the anatomical detail with the functional one, thus assessing the continuum atrio-valve-ventricle right; there is also a discussion about the role of cardiopulmonary testing associated with eco-stress for the evaluation of the right heart and functional reserve.

In the sixth chapter I have chosen to focus attention on the group of pathologies most frequently encountered, i.e., tricuspid insufficiency secondary to left cardiac pathology. This nosological entity needs a separate and punctual treatment with its physiological and pathophysiological premises, the role of ventricular interdependence, pulmonary hypertension and mitral and aortic pathology.

In the seventh chapter it is the turn of the infectivologist who presents the causes, diagnostics and indications for the treatment of endocarditis on tricuspid valve; the treatment is complex and multidisciplinary, requiring an approach for which is invoked in recent guidelines the formation of an endocarditis team such is its complexity.

In chapter eight, the role of the tricuspid valve in the population of the adult congenital patient is illustrated with excellent and necessary synthesis. It is of great interest, in fact, that on the one hand patients with congenital heart disease have reached adulthood with the sequelae of the basic pathology, perhaps involving the tricuspid valve, or develop a functional pathology due to congenital heart disease or a consequent degenerative pathology of other valves due to aging.

Also, tumours can be localized at the level of the right, primitive and secondary sections, such as to involve both primitively and for continuity the tricuspid valve; the treatment, entrusted to the anatomo-pathologist, focuses on the most frequent nosological entities and on the anatomical-clinical correlates.

In the tenth chapter are proposed the indications and the medical management of tricuspid insufficiency and right decompensation conditions.

The tricuspid valve also plays an important role, together with the right ventricle in patients undergoing cardiac transplantation or the implantation of a ventricular circulation assistance system (LVAD). The debate addressed in the eleventh chapter is broad and concerns the need for evaluation of trichuspidal insufficiency, right heart and pre-implantation correction of valvular disease and its impact in this particular population of patients.

In the twelfth chapter I illustrate the role of surgery in the management of functional failure of the tricuspid valve; in this context I thought it appropriate to illustrate and demystify the most resistant concepts in the world of tricuspid surgery, that is, if and when to intervene, how to stratify the risk of the patient with associated pathology and especially isolated and finally what techniques and devices to adopt to offer the best results in the short and long term.

Finally, in the thirteenth chapter, let's take a look at what will be one of the possible scenarios of surgery on the tricuspid valve: the transcatheter option. This type of approach has the undoubted advantage of avoiding extracorporeal circulation and cardioplegic arrest of the heart; in particular, it would benefit all patients with a borderline right ventricle or dysfunction too severe for surgery but despite all seriously limited by symptoms. The reader will find interesting the development and technological applications adopted and in particular the pathophysiological principles on which they were developed and their application.

I would like to thank all the Authors who have dedicated time and passion to tricuspid valve pathology, which I believe should not be considered a minor topic with respect to the predominant mitral or aortic valve; moreover, compared to the left atrio-ventricular valve (mitral valve) it cannot be considered as a right-sided surrogate in terms of pathophysiology, but requires its own analysis and its own tailored treatment.

In: The Rediscovered Tricuspid Valve ISBN: 978-1-53616-098-7
Editor: Giacomo Bianchi

Chapter 1

The Tricuspid Valve: From the "Forgotten" Valve to the "Fulcrum" of the Right Heart Historical Perspective

Giacomo Bianchi*[*]*, MD, PhD
Adult Cardiac Surgery Department, Ospedale del Cuore,
Fondazione "G. Monasterio," Massa, Italy

Abstract

The current knowledge of the cardiovascular system has established itself over the centuries after a stagnation perpetrated by theoretical medicine that was based on a prevailing galenism until the Renaissance. Even after the beginning of anatomical medicine and surgical anatomy, the synthesis between life, circulatory motion and cardiovascular system was a late achievement, whose turning point is represented by the work of William Harvey. Subsequently, the fine understanding of the physiological and pathophysiological mechanisms, especially in the right heart and the role of the tricuspid valve, are to be considered very recent;

---

[*] Corresponding Author's E-mail: gbianchi@ftgm.it.

still ongoing, although the scientific evidence accumulates, is the debate about whether and when to operate the tricuspid valve, despite the general underestimation of the problem and the high human cost and resources that failure to treat means.

Keywords: history, tricuspid valve

Historical Perspective

> "Après avoir ouvert ce ventricule on y voit du premiere coup un corps membraneux fort mince, que l'anciens Anatomistes ont regardé comme trois valvules, qu'ils ont appellé triglossines. Ces valvules sont garnies par le bas, de plusieurs perits ligamens ronds, tendineux, qui s'inferent sur íc sommet de trois éminences de grosseur inégale, qu'on appelle colomnes charneuses."[1]

> "After opening this ventricle, we see at first sight a very thin membranous body, which the ancient Anatomists saw as three valves, which they called triglossines[2]. These valves are joined at the bottom with different ligamentous tendons, which are inserted on top of three eminences of unequal size, called colomnes charneuses."[3]

The current vision of the cardiovascular system has taken centuries to complete, remaining in a state of erroneous conception of the circulatory pathophysiology perpetrated essentially by Galen (Pergamum 129 - Rome 201 AD).

In the conception of Galen, the liver is the source of all veins and the main source of blood formation [1, 2]. Blood is distributed through the hepatic veins from the liver to the lower vena cava, the latter with its ramifications brings nourishment to all organs. In this centrifugal vision,

---

[1] Vieussens R "Traité nouveau de la structure et des causes du mouvement naturel du coeur". Oeuvres françoises de M. Vieussens dédiées a nosseigneurs des états de la province de Languedoc. Toulouse: Jean Guillemette, 1715.

[2] Literally "three tongues", a clear reference to the three valve leaflets that are attached to a hingeline and that unfold after the opening of the right ventricle.

[3] This term refers to the papillary muscles.

the blood is absorbed by the organs but does not have a centripetal phase, that is, once assimilated it is lost.

In the galenic view, the right sections of the heart have a dual function, that of ducting and refining the blood to the lungs for nourishment.

Galen conceives of an open type of circulation, since he ignores the process of oxygenation and the return of blood through the pulmonary veins in the left atrium. He thinks that the blood from the right ventricle passes through invisible pores to the left ventricle for the formation of the vital spirit [3]. No mention is made of the right atrio-ventricular valve and the relative half-moon. The galenic error of the pores of the interventriocular septum will keep Western medicine crystallized for a millennium, until the Renaissance, requiring in fact 10 centuries before his vision was challenged.

In the middle of the 13th century, Ibn al-Naif questioned Galen's theories in two cardinal points of the circulation: 1. he did not believe that there were pores in the interventricular septum and that the left ventricular filling implied the circulation of blood from the right ventricle through the pulmonary tree; 2. the function of the right ventricle was responsible for the preparation of the blood that was preparing for the pulmonary circulation, refining it, making it fit to mix with the air [4].

In a completely independent manner and without access to the Arab source, Servetus and Columbus only rediscovered the lung circulation in 16th Century. Both authors, however, remain obedient to Galen and say that only a part of the blood passes into the lung circulation, while most remains in the vena cava from which it departs centrifugally to the organs; the discovery, serves only to overcome the theory of the non-existent pores in the interventricular septum and to provide an explanation of the passage of blood from the right sections to those on the left.

In general, the Humanism prone to the anatomical investigation, if on the one hand it opens the door to progress, on the other it does not determine the fall of the galenic vision; the latter is endowed with such internal coherence and is so rooted and perpetrated for centuries that the new discoveries are only additions to the ancient system.

Only with William Harvey (Folkestone, April 1, 1578 - Roehampton, June 3, 1657) were the crystallized galenic conceptions on circulation broken down with the publication of the book "Exercitatio Anatomica De Motu Cordis et Sanguinis in Animalibus." In particular, with reference to our topic of interest, Harvey challenges, starting from anatomical observation, Galen's statement about the function of the right ventricle. Harvey wonders, in fact, why the Nature created the right ventricle for the sole purpose of feeding the lung; why if it receives, as Galen says, only a small portion of blood, the pulmonary artery is as large as the aorta that supplies systemic blood; why the Nature needed a ventricle to feed an organ? Harvey concludes that the lung receives blood under the pressure of the right ventricular contraction through the pulmonary artery and from it, through the pulmonary veins returns to the right atrium and is finally ejected into the systemic circulation by the left ventricle. Then Nature invented the right ventricle not to feed the lung but to push the blood through the lungs into the left ventricle.

What was the clinical correlate of a tricuspid pathology or at least how certain signs reflected this valve pathology required a significant evolution of medical and scientific reasoning?

In 1704, Homberg described in the autopsy report of a 35-year-old woman, asthmatic, an important dilatation of the cardiac cavities that were flaccid "like a bag of leather"; he attributed the cervical pulsation to the reflux of blood in the veins of the neck to each contraction of the heart. Thus, he was the first to suggest the association between right ventricular dysfunction, tricuspid insufficiency and high filling pressures of the right ventricle.

In 1715, Raymond Vieussens in his work "Traité nouveau de la structure et des causes du mouvement naturel du coeur" described the internal structure of the right ventricle and gave a detailed anatomy of the tricuspid valve and the pulmonary valve; however, his intention remained limited to the field of anatomy as such, without functional or surgical correlates (Figure 1).

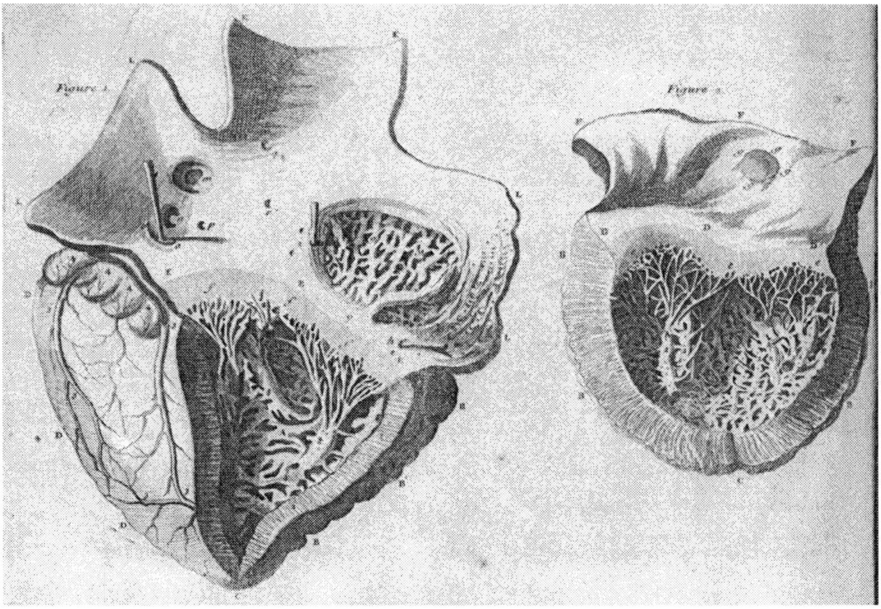

Figure 1. Table 10 of the "Traité nouveau de la structure et des causes du mouvement nature"; in the figure to the left of the reader (called Figure 1) the anatomical structures at the opening of the right atrium and ventricle are observed. In the figure on the right (called Figure 2) there is a greater focus on the right atrioventricular valve (called "triglossines" by the author), its leaflets and on the sub-valvular apparatus.

A few years later (1728), Lancisi described in the "Fifty-seventh proposition" of the "De motu cordis et aneurysmatibus" even more in detail the pathophysiology of the phenomenon: the pulsation of the neck veins comes from a dilated tricuspid valve associated with a right ventricle that is forced to push the blood both towards the pulmonary artery and retrograde towards the ostium of the caval veins.

However, this vision was questioned by Morgagni in 1769, who attributed the "sign of Lancisi" only to the overdistension of the right ventricle as described in the « Sedibus et Causis Morborum per Anatomen Indagatis."

Corvisart in the "Essai sur les maladies et les lésions organiques du coeur et des gros vaisseaux." condensed his knowledge of heart failure, describing it from a mechanical point of view and was also the first to describe the effort dyspnoea; in the observation n. 30, he impeccably described the turgidity of the face, neck and the prominent cyanosis of a 60-year-old man who had been hospitalised and was about to die. At the autopsy both atrioventricular valves demonstrated an important thickening (like cartilages, as described in the original text). Corvisart then focused his attention on the organic and functional causes of tricuspid valve disease.

The fusion of clinical observation, anatomy and pathophysiology in tricuspid pathology has required a very long gestation.

Observations such as that of the Dublin surgeon Robert Adams (1824) made some conceptual errors perpetrating over the years. Starting from cases in which it was recognized a marked pulmonary congestion, presumably also present a pulmonary hypertension, he was intrigued by the marked difference between the weakness of the systemic pulse and the strength of the precordial contractions deduced from the palpation. By disproving the presence of pulmonary hypertension, he developed a theory whereby the volume regurgitated by the tricuspid valve is the result of the portion of the right stroke volume that cannot be pushed into the lungs or accepted by the weakened left ventricle. This theory was based on the anatomical observations of John Hunter who had affirmed the weakness of the right structures of the heart compared to those of the left.

In an independent but concomitant way Thomas Wilkinson King of Guy's Hospital (London 1832) postulated the function of "safety valve" of the tricuspid in the right ventricle, identifying it as "life-saving" mechanism.

A pathophysiological legacy that would be perpetuated even a hundred years later in Mackenzie's iconic statement supported by Keith's anatomical authority, according to which the primary pathology of the valve was rare, while more frequent was valve regurgitation, so frequent that he wondered if the valve itself was capable of being properly continent.

Only with Laennec's invention of the stethoscope could the period between systole and diastole be defined first and then the murmur of insufficiency of the atrioventricular valve be described accurately.

Between 1866 and 1868 both Friedreich and Dorozier evaluated the presence of tricuspid insufficiency in congestive heart failure, thus characterizing a syndrome with venous distension, enlarged and pulsating liver, development of ascites, systolic breath of *centrum cordis* and distension of the veins of the neck.

The medical and surgical history of the right ventricle and its atrio-ventricular valve also present at the end of the XIXth and throughout the XXth centuries a troubled life, with experiments to assess the need for it, disconfirmations and rehabilitation at a structure necessary for the ventricular system.

In the 1940s in which more detailed studies on the function of the RV were performed. Experimental studies of RV cauterization did not lead to changes in systemic nor pulmonary artery pressure [5–7]; several studies conducted between 1950 and 1980 concluded that the RV was necessary for the maintenance of blood flow and life [8].

In 1982, Goldstein et al. demonstrated that RV myocardial infarction, using an animal model with intact pericardium, did lead to a reduction of cardiac output [9]. All the studies since then have shed light on the RV not just as a passive conduit for systemic venous return: the RV plays an important role in maintaining cardiac output in both health and disease.

Since the ventricle itself can be affected and can reflect its disease on the valve, one could argue that surgical research for tricuspid valve surgery should have been developed in a parallel fashion. This is not the case since it took a long time not only for the tricuspid valve to be recognized as a surgical target, but also the technology to operate on took a while before being present and widespread.

The first surgery on the tricuspid valve in the era of closed heart surgery took place two weeks after an initial mitral commissurotomy; the patient developed a major distension of the right appendage and atrial fibrillation. The tricuspid commissurotomy was performed by Trace et al. in May 1952 on a 24-year-old woman; the patient had a good recovery and the report was published two years later [10]. Combined mitral and tricuspid commissurotomy was also performed by Brofman in 1953 [11].

In 1967, Grondin et al. described the surgical treatment of the tricuspid valve pathology as a “challenge” [12]. Since mitral or aortic pathology often predominated over the tricuspid valve, it often remained neglected; in turn, the presence of ventricular dysfunction or the patient’s volemic state could affect the degree of tricuspid regurgitation and therefore depose or not for its surgical correction. It appears evident that this valve was poorly understood at the time and had probably been left undertreated more than necessary.

Tricuspid regurgitation, often secondary to left-sided heart pathology, is not rare and has a major impact on patients’ prognosis. The natural history of tricuspid regurgitation from flail leaflets without associated cardiovascular disease demonstrated an increased risk of atrial fibrillation, symptoms, heart failure, surgery, or death [13].

Being organic in origin or secondary to other diseases, the way in which surgeons began to treat tricuspid insufficiency was to start from the occurrence of annular dilatation and try to bring back to coaptation the leaflets, acting on the annulus ring itself.

Kay was the first author to apply a reconstructive surgical technique for TR [14] that consisted in creating a bicuspid valve consequent to an annular reduction and suture-based exclusion of the posterior leaflet. Although an intelligent and effective solution in the short term, the lack of stabilization of the anteroposterior commissure resulted in poor durability.

In 1972, De Vega introduced a sutured, non-annuloplasty technique, consisting in two rows of semi-circular sutures tied on both sides on pledgets over a 28- or 30-mm dilatator to avoid the purse string effect [15]. This method, quick relatively cheap and highly reproducible, became very popular and had several modifications over the years by some authors [16–18]. Although different in description, each of them aimed at overcoming an intrinsic limitation of the De Vega technique, that is the recurrence of insufficiency from distension of the suture, the so-called “guitar-string valve incompetence”.

The real turning point in the understanding of pathological changes in the tricuspid valve during pathological processes is attributable to Alain Carpentier, who in 1974 presented his vision of annular remodeling not only associated with a restrictive valve plastic, but also with a semi-rigid ring adapting to the cardiac cycle [19].

Duran pushed further this concept of « physiological motion" of the annulus introducing his flexible prosthetic ring in 1975.

More recent works have focused more on adjunctive techniques to reduce the TR since it correlates with patients' prognosis; some techniques are modifications of the correspective on the mitral valve, as the "Clover" technique, where the three margins of the tricuspid valve are sutured together along with a prosthetic ring [20]; other techniques address the tethering of the leaflets in advanced disease, like the augmentation of the anterior leaflet [21, 22].

In centuries of research on blood circulation, from the difficult understanding of the anatomical-clinical correlate of tricuspid insufficiency, after more than 50 years from the first surgical experience of tricuspid valve correction, it is still difficult to overcome the legacy of that tradition that wants the tricuspid valve as a secondary structure, intrinsically weak or even a benign epiphenomenon of heart disease.

The clinician, the surgeon, the researcher, often merged in the same figure, have to consider the tricuspid pathology a nosological entity in its own right. It is not an image in the mirror of the mitral pathology nor does it have the same pathophysiological mechanisms, even if correlated. The valve is the fulcrum of the entire pathology of the right heart. Extreme attention must be paid to the search for parameters that indicate the timing of intervention and its modalities, as well as the management of the underlying causes but also the natural history of the valve disease in its own right.

The modern approach is to increasingly consider atrial, ventricular, pulmonary and cardiac rhythm parameters integrated with right ventricular mechanics rather than the absolute degree of valvular insufficiency.

In this way it will be possible to intervene in an appropriate and effective way on the disease and to modify its natural history.

REFERENCES

[1] Galen, Singer C (1956) *Galen on Anatomical Procedures: Translation of the Surviving Books; with Introduction and Notes.* Wellcome Historical Medical Museum.

[2] Galen P, Lacy D (1978) *Galen on the Doctrines of Hippocrates and Plato*. Akademie Verlag, Berlin.

[3] West JB (2008) Ibn al-Nafis, the pulmonary circulation, and the Islamic Golden Age. *J Appl Physiol Bethesda Md* 1985 105:1877–1880.

[4] Haddad SI, Khairallah AA (1936) A forgotten chapter in the history of the circulation of the blood. *Ann Surg* 104:1–8.

[5] Starr I, Jeffers WA, Meade Jr RH (1943) The absence of conspicuous increments of venous pressure after severe damage to the right ventricle of the dog, with a discussion of the relation between clinical congestive failure and heart disease. *Am Heart J* 26:291–301.

[6] Bakos ACP (1950) The question of the function of the right ventricular myocardium: an experimental study. *Circulation* 1:724–732.

[7] Kagan A (1952) Dynamic responses of the right ventricle following extensive damage by cauterization. *Circulation* 5:816–823.

[8] Dell'Italia LJ (1991) The right ventricle: anatomy, physiology, and clinical importance. *Curr Probl Cardiol* 16:653–720.

[9] Goldstein JA, Vlahakes GJ, Verrier ED, Schiller NB, Tyberg JV, Ports TA, Parmley WW, Chatterjee K (1982) The role of right ventricular systolic dysfunction and elevated intrapericardial pressure in the genesis of low output in experimental right ventricular infarction. *Circulation* 65:513–522.

[10] Trace HD, Bailey CP, Wendkos MH (1954) Tricuspid valve commissurotomy with a one-year follow-up. *Am Heart J* 47:613–618.

[11] Brofman B (1953) Right auriculoventricular pressure gradients with special reference to tricuspid stenosis. In: J. Lab. Clin. Med. *Mosby-*

Year Book Inc 11830 Westline Industrial Dr, St Louis, MO 63146-3318, pp 789–790.

[12] Grondin P, Lepage G, Castonguay Y, Meere C (1967) The tricuspid valve: a surgical challenge. *J Thorac Cardiovasc Surg* 53:7–20.

[13] Messika-Zeitoun D, Thomson H, Bellamy M, Scott C, Tribouilloy C, Dearani J, Tajik AJ, Schaff H, Enriquez-Sarano M (2004) Medical and surgical outcome of tricuspid regurgitation caused by flail leaflets. *J Thorac Cardiovasc Surg* 128:296–302.

[14] Kay JH, Maselli-Campagna G, Tsuji KK (1965) Surgical treatment of tricuspid insufficiency. *Ann Surg* 162:53–58.

[15] De Vega N (1972) La anuloplastica selective, regulable y permanente. *Rev Esp Cardiol* 555–556.

[16] Cabrol C (1972) Valvular annuloplasty. A new method. *Nouv Presse Med* 1:1366.

[17] Antunes MJ, Girdwood RW (1983) Tricuspid annuloplasty: a modified technique. *Ann Thorac Surg* 35:676–678.

[18] Revuelta JM, Garcia-Rinaldi R (1989) Segmental tricuspid annuloplasty: a new technique. *J Thorac Cardiovasc Surg* 97:799–801.

[19] Carpentier A, Deloche A, Hanania G, Forman J, Sellier P, Piwnica A, Dubost C, McGoon DC (1974) Surgical management of acquired tricuspid valve disease. *J Thorac Cardiovasc Surg* 67:53–65.

[20] Lapenna E, Bonis MD, Verzini A, Canna GL, Ferrara D, Calabrese MC, Taramasso M, Alfieri O (2010) The clover technique for the treatment of complex tricuspid valve insufficiency: midterm clinical and echocardiographic results in 66 patients. *Eur J Cardiothorac Surg* 37:1297–1303.

[21] Dreyfus GD, Raja SG, John Chan KM (2008) Tricuspid leaflet augmentation to address severe tethering in functional tricuspid regurgitation. *Eur J Cardio-Thorac Surg Off J Eur Assoc Cardio-Thorac Surg* 34:908–910.

[22] Solinas M, Bianchi G, Glauber M (2013) Easy and reproducible technique to address tricuspid valve regurgitation with patch augmentation. *J Card Surg* 28:638–640.

In: The Rediscovered Tricuspid Valve ISBN: 978-1-53616-098-7
Editor: Giacomo Bianchi

Chapter 2

THE FUNCTIONAL ANATOMY AND PATHOLOGY OF THE TRICUSPID VALVE: MORPHOGENESIS, NORMAL AND PATHOLOGICAL ANATOMY

Giacomo Bianchi[1,*], MD, PhD
and Angela Pucci[2], MD, PhD
[1]Adult Cardiac Surgery Department, Ospedale del Cuore,
Fondazione "G. Monasterio," Massa, Italy
[2]Dept. Of Anatomic Pathology, Pisa University Hospital, Massa, Italy

ABSTRACT

The tricuspid valve has a complex morphogenesis, orchestrated by a dense network of molecular signals. It intersects intimately with the cardiac morphogenesis. The understanding of it lays the foundations for the study of pathological processes and primitive forms of valvulopathy. However, it is also the key to understanding the functional anatomy that

* Corresponding Author's E-mail: gbianchi@ftgm.it.

becomes clinical anatomy with its related pathophysiological and surgical anatomy where interventional treatment is necessary.

Keywords: functional anatomy, morphogenesis, valvular pathology

Introduction

The systematic study of the right atrioventricular valve, or tricuspid valve, is fascinating and complex for the context in which it develops and operates, namely the particular geometry of the right ventricle, its anatomical relationship with other cardiac structures and its function. It is clear that for both the clinician and the cardiac surgeon the understanding of the mechanisms of valve disease and the morpho-functional bases for its repair cannot be separated from the knowledge of embryogenesis, of the components of normality, the normal and finally pathological variants of the tricuspid valve.

Tricuspid Valve Morphogenesis

Structural Components

Several components represent the building blocks of the tricuspid valve during morphogenesis: the extracellular matrix (ECM), the endothelial valve cells and the interstitial endothelial cells.

In the ECM a dense network of collagen fibers (type I, type II and V) interacts with other fibers and cells in the *fibrosa*; in the *spongiosa* the proteoglycans and glycosaminoglycans (GAG; hyaluronic acid, chondroitin-sulphates 4 and 6 and decorin) act as a buffer to resist the mechanical deformations of stretching and torsion; the very fine *pars atrialis* is composed of elastin and collagen with a radial orientation of the fibers themselves.

The ECM is not, however, a mere physical support for cell growth, but a biologically active structure with mechanical and humoral signals. Valve cells are linked to the ECM by local adhesion molecules such as actin filaments or hemidesmosomes, which in turn are linked to intermediate filaments such as keratin. Finally, integrins regulate the interaction with the ECM through the extra-cellular domains of GAG and laminine associated with fibronectin. In addition, hyaluronic acid and decorin can act as regular humors by seizing growth factors and receptors.

Valve endothelial cells (VECs) form a single layer of endothelial cells in continuity with the endocardium and endothelium [1]. They are morphologically different from vascular endothelial cells and respond differently to shear stress; in fact, they are oriented perpendicularly to it, regardless of the orientation of the ECM [2]. VECs have multiple physiological roles, such as mediating platelet aggregation, inflammation, fibroblast contraction and migration, and valve mechanics. In addition, in response to the damage, they may encounter EMT [3] and replace the pool of interstitial valve cells (VICs).

The latter (VICs) are a heterogeneous population of smooth muscle cells, fibroblasts and myofibroblasts interspersed between layers of ECM.

VICs are highly plastic and can undergo transformation into smooth muscle cells [4]. Each of these components has well-defined homeostatic roles: fibroblasts produce most of the ECM, while smooth muscle cells secrete both metalloprotease (MMPs) and their tissue inhibitors (TIMPs). During alterations of the mechanical load, the VICs respond by increasing tissue rigidity through the expression of active a-smooth muscles and a remodeling of the ECM in a fibrotic sense [5]; in turn, the feedback is completed with a modulation through the stiffness of the ECM on the biochemical response of the VICs.

Cardiac Development with Reference to the Right Atrioventricular Valve

Early Cardiac Development

The heart tube is derived from the first heart field (FHF) of the splanchnic mesoderm and contributes to the formation of the cardiac precursors of the atria, the atrioventricular canal (AVC) and the left ventricle [6]. At stage E9.0, the heart tube is folded clockwise with a posterior positioning of the atrium [7]. The cells of the pharyngeal mesenchyme known as the second heart field (SHF) migrate to elongate the heart in a polar sense; on the arterial pole they will give rise to the outflow tract (OFT), the right ventricle (RV) and the interventricular septum (IVS) [8, 9]; on the venous pole they contribute to the formation of atria and the interatrial septum through the AV septal complex [10].

Patterning of Cardiac Valve Territory

The only regions responsible for valve formation in humans are AVC and OFT. Endocardial bearings (ECs) are formed in these regions through tissue patterning and EMT. The morphogenetic program is closely linked to the mechanical forces produced by local hemodynamics [11, 12]. At stage E9.5 at OFT and AV level there is a proteoglycan-rich swelling of the ECM [13, 14]; the next day a subgroup of endocranial cells of the OFT and AV pads meet EMT and migrate within the cardiac jelly [13, 14].

The regulation is entrusted to a complex and articulated cytokine network: EMT is orchestrated by bone morphogenic proteins (BMPs), transforming growth factor beta (TGF-b) and Notch [15–18], whose beginning and end signal is given to the vascular endothelial growth factor (VEGF) [19–21]; the signaling of ErbB/SHP-2/NF-1/Ras promotes mesenchymal migration in cardiac jelly, proliferation and expansion of ECs mesenchyme [22–24].

Furthermore, the ECM itself is a regulator of EMT through hyaluronan synthase 2 (Has2), since high molecular weight hyaluronic acid (HA) on the one hand promotes EMT by activating ErbB2-ErbB3 receptors, and on the other hand in its depolymerized form limits the delimitation and transformation of endocardial cells [25, 26].

Cardiac Valve Morphogenesis

At stage E10.5, EMT ceases in AVC; the major ECs (upper/superior and lower/inferior) constitute the bulk of the mesenchyme that occupies the lumen of AVC. The major cushions take part in the formation of the mesenchymal complex AV, contributing to the formation of the aortic leaflet (anterior) of the mitral valve and the septal leaflet of the tricuspid valve [10].

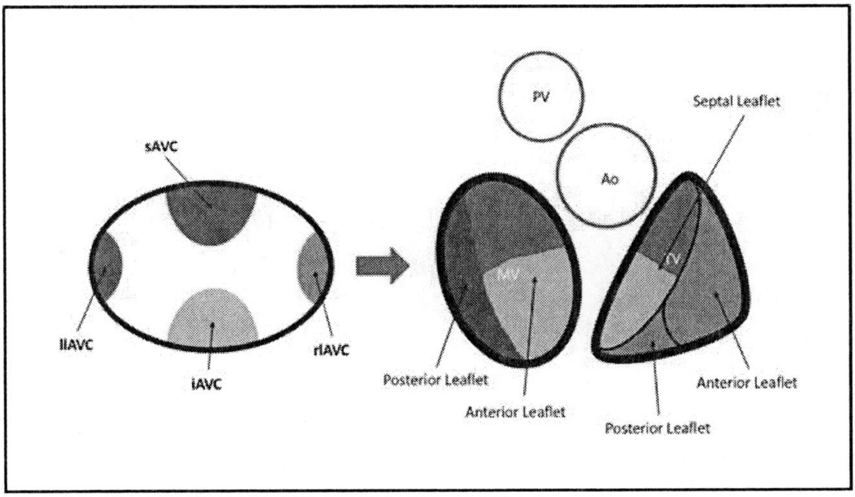

Figure 1. Contribution of each endocardial cushion to the formation of atrio-ventricular valves. sAVC: superior atrio-ventricular cushion; iAVC: inferior atrio-ventricular cushion; llAVC: left-lateral atrio-ventricular cushion; rlAVC: right-lateral cushion.

The lateral cushion behave differently, do not fuse and do not participate in the formation of the mesenchymal complex AV; instead, the right-lateral cushion participates in the formation of the antero-superior and posterior leaflet of the tricuspid valve, while the left-lateral cushion gives rise to the mural leaflet of the mitral valve [10] (Figure 1).

In the atrioventricular valves it is possible to trace the cell line of the different components through special markings. The mesenchyme of the major bearings is formed by endothelial and endocranial cells almost exclusively derived from endocardial EMT [10, 27]. Atrio-ventricular fibrous continuity, valve leaflets and tendon chordae are derived from the endocardium [28, 29]. The fibrous skeleton of the heart derives from epicardial cells (EPDCs) that populate the mesenchyme of the AV valves after EMT [10, 30]; in particular, in the tricuspidal and mitral mural leaflet, EPDCs constitute the majority of the mesenchyme.

The cells derived from the cranial neural crest (CNCCs), on the other hand, at E12.5 have been found almost exclusively in the septal leaflet of the tricuspid valve and in the anterior (aortic) leaflet of the mitral valve; these cells persist in the septal leaflet of the tricuspid even after birth [31].

Finally, AVC cardiomyocytes contribute to the development of the mural and posterior leaflets of the tricuspid; they are also present at the atrial edge of the annulus fibrosus, thus contributing to electrical isolation between the atrium and the ventricle [32].

From E11.5 onwards, CEs expand under the impulse of Bmp/TGF-b, EGF, Nf1/rad and Wnt [33–37] and mesenchymal-specific transcription factors [33, 38]. The fusion of the ECs leads to the subtraction of the left and right ventricular inlets.

In the late phase of valvulogenesis, the septal leaflet of the tricuspid remains in contact with the interventricular septum until delamination occurs at E17.5 [28, 32, 39]; MV and TV wall leaflets are supported by the ventricular myocardium; as the heart grows and the leaflets lengthen in the lumen, thin bands of muscle remain attached to the leaflet; a process of apoptosis makes the leaflets mobile and causes the remnants of the endocardium to form the tendon chordae and papillary muscles [28, 29].

In the final phase, the hemodynamic stimulus leads to the formation of VICs from undifferentiated mesenchyme [40, 41]; the ECM also undergoes remodeling, in a longer process that takes place in the late gestation phase and lasts after birth [18, 42–45].

Between E15.5 and E18.5 there is a process of "condensation," i.e., an increase in the cellularity of the AV leaflets [18]. The alignment of the ECM is guided by hemodynamic stress starting from the interaction with the endothelium [46]; after birth, the increase in the length of the valve leaflets is due to the traction on the tendon chordae of rapidly growing ventricles.

From an ultrastructural point of view, collagen fibrils are densely aggregated in areas with more hemodynamic stress, orchestrated by "*periostin,*" which blocks the differentiation of mesenchyme in other cell types, such as cardiomyocytes; in particular, this process is extremely active at the level of AV valves and their support apparatus [47, 48].

The coordinated action of ECM proteases on the one hand favors cell migration and proliferation, while on the other hand it can subvert the structure of the valve, such as in myxomatous degeneration where the presence of loose collagen, increased proteoglycans and alteration of fiber orientation are observed [43, 49, 50], associated with the aberrant expression of early mesenchymal markers, to be related to reactivation of a fetal transcription program [51, 52].

The Normal Tricuspid Valve

Components of the Tricuspid Valve

The tricuspid valve is a complex of different structures that contribute, operating in sync, to the opening during the diastole and to the closing in systole. These structures are represented by the valve leaflets, tendon chordae, papillary muscles and the annular attachment at the atrio-ventricular junction.

The tricuspid valve has three leaflets and, although their number has been questioned and in a study reported that the leaflets were actually two [53]; observation of the valve itself in the open position can be misleading and lead to this conclusion, but if observed in the closed position, the appearance is always that of a clovered structure: each part is suspended in a relatively circular annulus, supported by a completely muscular orifice [54].

In this regard, the annulus is a peculiar structure with interesting characteristics. At a macroscopic analysis both in vivo and on an anatomical sample, the tricuspidal annulus seems to demarcate the junction between the atrial and right ventricular myocardium with the interposed valve leaflets.

The reality is that although you have the impression of a rigid structure at this level, the leaflets are attached to a poorly formed fibrous ring and not as outlined as in the mitral valve [55].

At the level of the annulus, the atrial musculature overlaps very little with the "pars atrialis" of the leaflet, while the larger part is separated by offshoots of fibro-adipose tissue in which the right coronary artery and the coronary veins run. The connective tissue of the leaflet, on its side, is deeply united to the subendocardial tissue; it is united by merging with the peri-valvular connective tissue to create a triangular structure in section that constitutes the so-called "annulus."

The tricuspid orifice is larger than the mitral one, with a circumference between 8.7 and 15.5 cm and an area of 21.0 ± 1.1 cm^2 (range 14.5-35.1 cm^2) [56].

The annulus of the tricuspid valve is positioned vertically in an anatomical position. The structure is not bidimensional and uniplanar, but with a precise three-dimensional arrangement that is appreciable when the heart is opened along the acute margin: the attachment of the leaflets to the annulus is not at the same level [57].

Tricuspid Leaflets and Commissures

The leaflets of the right atrioventricular valve, or tricuspid valve, vary in number (in one study only 62% had 3 distinct leaflets), while they invariably have three closing lines, but have distinct zones and layers [58] (Figure 2).

The *basal zone* is the part of the leaflet that is attached to the annulus at the atrioventricular junction. In this area, the leaflet receives innervation and vascularization from nearby structures. The *clear zone* is the largest portion of the leaflet, occupying two-thirds of the leaflet, from the basal zone to the free margin. It is fine and translucent. The *rough area* is found in the portion of the margin and in the zone of insertions.

From a histological point of view, 4 zones can be distinguished: atrialis, spongiosa, fibrosa and ventricularis. The *atrialis* layer consists of elastin and collagen fibers covered with endothelium; it is the area with the highest number of elastic fibers. It has the function of dissipating energy at the time of opening and closing the valve.

Spongiosa is rich in ECM (proteoglycans, glycosaminoglycans, elastic fibers); due to its composition it is richly hydrated and constitutes a good part of the free margin. It has a shock absorber function. The fibrous pars, rich in collagen, has the task of giving the valve a resistance to tensile loads. Finally, the *pars ventricularis* is nothing more than a continuous sheet of endothelium that covers the elastic fibers and collagen.

In view of the orientation of the heart in normal anatomy, the valve leaflets are called anterosuperior, septal and inferior. The nomenclature of the leaflets in literature is not uniform; the anterosuperior leaflet is often called also anterior, the inferior leaflet called also posterior or mural.

The tricuspid leaflets do not all lie on the same level [59] and their attack is nonplanar [60].

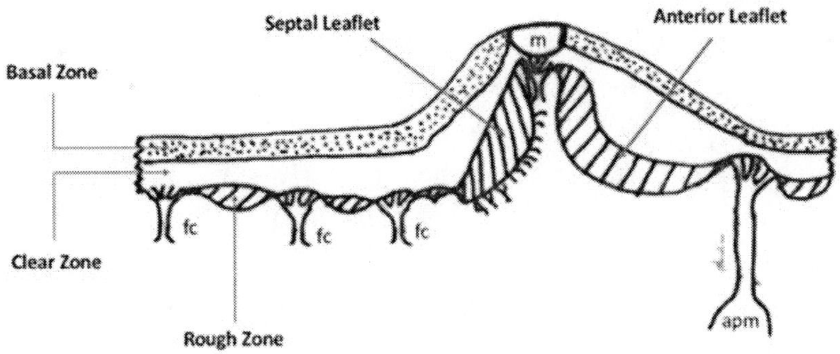

Figure 2. Schematics of tricuspid valve opened through the posterior leaflet: the three basal, clear and rough zones are depicted. fc: fan-shaped chordae; m: membranous septum; apm: anterior papillary muscle. Note that chordae for the septal leaflet are depicted as small delaminations from the myocardium.

In particular, the University of Toronto group recognized that the posterior (lower) leaflet attachment and the postero-septal half of the septal leaflet are horizontal and 15 mm lower than the maximum valve attachment point; the highest point is at the level of the middle portion of the membranous septum to the antero-septal commissure; finally, in the middle of the septal leaflet, the leaflet and the hinge-line have an increase in the angle of about 30° to reach the antero-septal commissure [57].

From an atrial vision, the three leaflets delimit a triangular orifice; each of them has differences that can be postponed, which helps the characterization and differentiation.

The *anterior* leaflet (infundibular, lateral, upper) has a semicircular shape, in some cases even quadrangular, has a smooth or indented margin of coaptation (Silver 1971); it is the largest and widest, extending like a curtain for half of the free wall of the right ventricle (from the infundibular region of outflow to the lower part of the right ventricle). It contributes for the most part to the continence of the valve [61].

The *posterior* leaflet (marginal, dorsal or inferior) has many indentations or clefts that give it the appearance of multiple scallops. In the clefts, tendon chords with a fan-like appearance are inserted. Anatomically, this leaflet occupies the lower portion of the valve and originates from the diaphragmatic wall of the right ventricle.

Of all tricuspid leaflets, the *septal* (medial) leaflet is the most anatomically and pathophysiologically complex. It occupies the smallest portion of the annulus; the tendon chordae attach directly to the septal myocardium and partly to the posterior wall of the right heart; in the middle of the leaflet, its attachments converge at the base of the heart, to reach the antero-septal commissure at the level of the membranous septum. Moreover, it is located more apically than the other leaflets; in a view of the heart in 4 chambers it is possible to see how on the plane passing between the membranous septum and the septal leaflet, the tricuspid valve appears lower than the mitral valve.

In addition to the normal indentures, the tricuspid valve also has some of them deeper, called commissures, which identify the transition zone between the valve leaflets. The *antero-septal commissure* is the easiest to identify; it is in fact adjacent to the membrane pars of the interventricular septum. There is usually a continuity between the anterior and septal leaflet: a part of the valve leaflet extends for about 1-5 mm in depth; in most cases there is not a real transition between one leaflet and another, but a continuum between the two leaflets [56]. The *anterior-posterior commissure* is easy to identify, since it is crossed almost invariably by the anterior papillary muscle. *Posteroseptal commissure* is identified by considering the free margin of the septal leaflet which is notched with respect to the posterior leaflet whose margin is smooth.

Tendinous Chords and Papillary Muscles

The elongated and fibrous tendon chordae are the key structures that connect the papillary muscles with the leaflets. The systematization of the tendinous chordae in relation to their origin and attack on the leaflets differs among researchers and has generated wide debate.

About 170 tendinous chordae are present for each tricuspid valve, with a higher density in women and at the level of the septal leaflet in both sexes [56].

In his seminal work, Silver et al. recognize 5 types of tendinous chordae: *fan-shaped, free-edge chordae, deep chordae, rough zone chordae* and *basal chordae* [57]. Approximately 50% of the chordae are distributed on the free margin, the remainder on the ventricular and basal surface of the leaflet.

Although the "fan-shaped" chordae are identified by Silver as pathognomonic of the commissures, this statement has been questioned more recently, as it is not the only distinctive feature nor exclusive of the commissures [56]. The anatomical-functional characteristic of the fan-shaped chordae is that they connect the leaflets, favor their separation during the diastole and increase the area of commissural coaptation during the systole [62]. Therefore, they are also called interleaflet chordae and have multiple connections to adjacent leaflets. A more modern view of the tendinous chordae, in fact, identifies only two systems, the interleaflet chordae and the leaflet chordae.

Leaflets chordae include tendon chordae from the rough area that fit onto the ventricular surface of the leaflet. Thicker chordae are sometimes also called strut chordae because they also support most of the mechanical stress during the cardiac cycle. Deep chordae fit onto the ventricular face of the leaflet at the level of the rough and clear zone. Leaflet chordae that fit at the free margin are simply called free-edge chordae.

The leaflets chordae originate from the papillary muscles with an almost constant pattern: from the medial papillary muscle (also known as conal or Lancisi's muscle) or from a small area adjacent to the membranous septum for the septal portion of the anterior leaflet; from the prominent anterior papillary muscle for the posterior half of the anterior leaflet and the anterior half of the posterior leaflet; from the group of posterior papillaries for the posterior half of the posterior leaflet and a small portion of the septal leaflet; finally, the septal leaflet is served almost exclusively by direct or single chordae from the septal myocardium.

The insertion pattern on the leaflet is also constant: direct (as in the case of the septal leaflet), radial or arched (anterior and posterior leaflet) and fan-shaped (cleft and commissure).

The anterior papillary muscle is the largest of the papillary muscles; it is composed of distinct muscle fibers with multiple heads, usually resulting in bifid or tripartite. Sometimes more papillary muscles converge in it, determining the presence of a single dominant papillary, surrounded by minor papillaries. In general, the anterior papillary muscle is born from the moderating band after it has passed through the right ventricular cavity; specifically, it may depart from the middle portion or shortly before it connects with the right ventricular free wall [61].

The lower papillary muscle supports the mixture of lower and septal leaflets; very often it is not identifiable as a stand-alone structure, but rather consists of multiple papillary heads serving the same area.

The medial papillary muscle is born from the postero-caudal portion of the septum-marginal trabecula (or moderating band); the base of the medial papillary muscle is an important anatomical landmark as it marks the entrance of the right branch of the beam into the ventricular myocardium. Fan-shaped interleaflet chordae for antero-septal commissure originate from it; although it is a papillary with a single head, it may be accompanied by multiple others with cordial insertions for the anterior and septal leaflet in the vicinity of the commissure [61].

The Pathological Tricuspid Valve

Tricuspid Valve Regurgitation

The fact that the dysfunction of the tricuspid valve causes an alteration of the blood circulation has been known since ancient times [63]. The most known alteration in function and related to a pathological picture is undoubtedly valvular insufficiency.

The causes of this valve regurgitation can be classified as degenerative and functional. The degenerative causes can be traced back to problems related to the valve itself, i.e., to the leaflets or the tensor apparatus (tendon chordae and papillary muscles); the functional forms include dilation of the right atrial and ventricular chamber.

Degenerative causes include structural problems such as leaflet prolapse, leaflet dysplasia, myxomatous valves, papillary fibroelastoma, rheumatic disease, endocarditis, carcinoid disease, iatrogenic lesions such as pacemaker implantation lesions in which the septal leaflet may be perforated or degenerated following the formation of peri-catheter fibrosis, as well as damage to the leaflets or subvalvular apparatus in endomyocardial biopsies. In functional forms we find atrial enlargement for example in primitive forms of atrial fibrillation [64], in right ventricular dilatation from primitive or secondary pulmonary hypertension [65, 66] or dilated cardiomyopathy and in chronic ischemic forms or in right ventricular infarction.

Although beyond the scope of this text, which takes into account the role of the tricuspid valve in adults, an important mention is reserved for congenital heart disease and in particular the most common form of congenital pathology of the valve, namely the Ebstein anomaly. From a developmental point of view, there is an incomplete delimitation of the septal and inferior (mural) leaflets from the ventricular myocardium; thus, the hingelines of the two leaflets are located far below the atrioventricular plane. This apical displacement of the leaflets may be of varying degrees: in mild forms, this offset is difficult to recognize, while in severe forms the leaflets appear as dystrophic and poorly delineated compared to the ventricular myocardium or may be absent. The right ventricle is then discounted and associated with a variable degree of valvular regurgitation.

Tricuspid Valve Stenosis

In tricuspid stenosis, one or more components of the valve are malformed or subverted as a result of a pathological process. Ultimately, there is a reduction in the size of the valve orifice and an obstacle to flow, often in conjunction with some degree of regurgitation.

The acquired forms may include healed infectious processes characterized by retracting fibrosis, sometimes perforations are also present in the context that result in regurgitation of varying degrees; in active infections, the endocarditic mass can be so voluminous as to end intermittent stenosis of the valve. Tricuspid stenosis secondary to rheumatic disease is the most common form in children. From a macroscopic point of view, the valve presents commissure fusion, cord shortening, as well as reduced motility and leaflet excursion; in the final analysis, the valve is both stenotic and regurgitating.

A hint at congenital forms: malformed tricuspid valves can be found as an isolated form concerning an altered development of the leaflets or subvalvular apparatus, as well as being associated with congenital cardiac malformations. The most extreme form is atresia of the tricuspid valve, where often there is no hint of valve formation and the heart is univentricular, where the only way of outflow to the venous return is through broad interatrial communication. Intermediate forms of tricuspidal stenosis are associated with diseases of the right efflux, as in the case of pulmonary stenosis/pulmonary atresia; in these congenital malformations, the valve consists of rudimentary leaflets and subvalvular apparatus; often stenosis is associated with a variable degree of valvular regurgitation.

CONCLUSION

The understanding of the functional anatomy of the tricuspid valve starts from the fine knowledge of its morphogenesis; on it depends not only the entire spectrum of primary pathology that can present itself to the clinician, but also the anatomical substrate.

The efforts of the cardiologist and surgeon are focused on the knowledge of the latter, both in the visualization of the mechanisms of disease, on the pathological substrate but also on the normal anatomy. On the latter is based all the current action but also all the research for the development and implementation of new techniques and devices for the surgical and interventional treatment of valvulopathy.

REFERENCES

[1] Tao G, Kotick JD, Lincoln J (2012) Heart valve development, maintenance, and disease: the role of endothelial cells. *Curr Top Dev Biol* 100:203–232.

[2] Butcher JT, Nerem RM (2006) Valvular endothelial cells regulate the phenotype of interstitial cells in co-culture: effects of steady shear stress. *Tissue Eng* 12:905–915.

[3] Bischoff J, Aikawa E (2011) Progenitor cells confer plasticity to cardiac valve endothelium. *J Cardiovasc Transl Res* 4:710–719.

[4] Rabkin-Aikawa E, Farber M, Aikawa M, Schoen FJ (2004) Dynamic and reversible changes of interstitial cell phenotype during remodeling of cardiac valves. *J Heart Valve Dis* 13:841–847.

[5] Weston MW, Yoganathan AP (2001) Biosynthetic activity in heart valve leaflets in response to in vitro flow environments. *Ann Biomed Eng* 29:752–763.

[6] Buckingham M, Meilhac S, Zaffran S (2005) Building the mammalian heart from two sources of myocardial cells. *Nat Rev Genet* 6:826–835.

[7] Männer J (2009) The anatomy of cardiac looping: a step towards the understanding of the morphogenesis of several forms of congenital cardiac malformations. *Clin Anat N Y N* 22:21–35.

[8] Zaffran S, Kelly RG, Meilhac SM, Buckingham ME, Brown NA (2004) Right ventricular myocardium derives from the anterior heart field. *Circ Res* 95:261–268.

[9] Verzi MP, McCulley DJ, De Val S, Dodou E, Black BL (2005) The right ventricle, outflow tract, and ventricular septum comprise a restricted expression domain within the secondary/anterior heart field. *Dev Biol* 287:134–145.

[10] Snarr BS, Kern CB, Wessels A (2008) Origin and fate of cardiac mesenchyme. *Dev Dyn Off Publ Am Assoc Anat* 237:2804–2819.

[11] Egorova AD, Khedoe PPSJ, Goumans M-JTH, Yoder BK, Nauli SM, ten Dijke P, Poelmann RE, Hierck BP (2011) Lack of primary cilia primes shear-induced endothelial-to-mesenchymal transition. *Circ Res* 108:1093–1101.

[12] Riem Vis PW, Kluin J, Sluijter JPG, van Herwerden LA, Bouten CVC (2011) Environmental regulation of valvulogenesis: implications for tissue engineering. *Eur J Cardio-Thorac Surg Off J Eur Assoc Cardio-Thorac Surg* 39:8–17.

[13] Eisenberg LM, Markwald RR (1995) Molecular regulation of atrioventricular valvuloseptal morphogenesis. *Circ Res* 77:1–6.

[14] Person AD, Klewer SE, Runyan RB (2005) Cell biology of cardiac cushion development. *Int Rev Cytol* 243:287–335.

[15] Yamagishi T, Ando K, Nakamura H (2009) Roles of TGFbeta and BMP during valvulo-septal endocardial cushion formation. *Anat Sci Int* 84:77–87.

[16] Lencinas A, Tavares ALP, Barnett JV, Runyan RB (2011) Collagen gel analysis of epithelial-mesenchymal transition in the embryo heart: an in vitro model system for the analysis of tissue interaction, signal transduction, and environmental effects. *Birth Defects Res Part C Embryo Today Rev* 93:298–311.

[17] de la Pompa JL, Epstein JA (2012) Coordinating tissue interactions: Notch signaling in cardiac development and disease. *Dev Cell* 22:244–254.

[18] Kruithof BPT, Krawitz SA, Gaussin V (2007) Atrioventricular valve development during late embryonic and postnatal stages involves condensation and extracellular matrix remodeling. *Dev Biol* 302:208–217.

[19] Dor Y, Camenisch TD, Itin A, Fishman GI, McDonald JA, Carmeliet P, Keshet E (2001) A novel role for VEGF in endocardial cushion formation and its potential contribution to congenital heart defects. *Dev Camb Engl* 128:1531–1538.

[20] Chang CP, Neilson JR, Bayle JH, Gestwicki JE, Kuo A, Stankunas K, Graef IA, Crabtree GR (2004) A field of myocardial-endocardial NFAT signaling underlies heart valve morphogenesis. *Cell* 118:649–663.

[21] Stankunas K, Ma GK, Kuhnert FJ, Kuo CJ, Chang C-P (2010) VEGF signaling has distinct spatiotemporal roles during heart valve development. *Dev Biol* 347:325–336.

[22] Yutzey KE, Colbert M, Robbins J (2005) Ras-related signaling pathways in valve development: ebb and flow. *Physiol Bethesda Md* 20:390–397.

[23] Iwamoto R, Mekada E (2006) ErbB and HB-EGF signaling in heart development and function. *Cell Struct Func*t 31:1–14.

[24] Sanchez-Soria P, Camenisch TD (2010) ErbB signaling in cardiac development and disease. *Semin Cell Dev Biol* 21:929–935.

[25] Camenisch TD, Schroeder JA, Bradley J, Klewer SE, McDonald JA (2002) Heart-valve mesenchyme formation is dependent on hyaluronan-augmented activation of ErbB2-ErbB3 receptors. *Nat Med* 8:850–855.

[26] Rodgers LS, Lalani S, Hardy KM, Xiang X, Broka D, Antin PB, Camenisch TD (2006) Depolymerized hyaluronan induces vascular endothelial growth factor, a negative regulator of developmental epithelial-to-mesenchymal transformation. *Circ Res* 99:583–589.

[27] Rivera-Feliciano J, Lee KH, Kong SW, Rajagopal S, Ma Q, Springer Z, Izumo S, Tabin CJ, Pu WT (2006) Development of heart valves requires Gata4 expression in endothelial-derived cells. *Dev Camb Engl* 133:3607–3618.

[28] de Lange FJ, Moorman AFM, Anderson RH, Männer J, Soufan AT, de Gier-de Vries C, Schneider MD, Webb S, van den Hoff MJB, Christoffels VM (2004) Lineage and morphogenetic analysis of the cardiac valves. *Circ Res* 95:645–654.

[29] Lincoln J, Alfieri CM, Yutzey KE (2004) Development of heart valve leaflets and supporting apparatus in chicken and mouse embryos. *Dev Dyn Off Publ Am Assoc Anat* 230:239–250.

[30] Gittenberger-de Groot AC, Bartram U, Oosthoek PW, Bartelings MM, Hogers B, Poelmann RE, Jongewaard IN, Klewer SE (2003) Collagen type VI expression during cardiac development and in human fetuses with trisomy 21. *Anat Rec A Discov Mol Cell Evol Biol* 275:1109–1116.

[31] Nakamura T, Colbert MC, Robbins J (2006) Neural crest cells retain multipotential characteristics in the developing valves and label the cardiac conduction system. *Circ Res* 98:1547–1554.

[32] Gaussin V, Morley GE, Cox L, et al. (2005) Alk3/Bmpr1a receptor is required for development of the atrioventricular canal into valves and annulus fibrosus. *Circ Res* 97:219–226.

[33] Gitler AD, Zhu Y, Ismat FA, Lu MM, Yamauchi Y, Parada LF, Epstein JA (2003) Nf1 has an essential role in endothelial cells. *Nat Genet* 33:75–79.

[34] Iwamoto R, Yamazaki S, Asakura M, et al. (2003) Heparin-binding EGF-like growth factor and ErbB signaling is essential for heart function. *Proc Natl Acad Sci USA* 100:3221–3226.

[35] Jackson LF, Qiu TH, Sunnarborg SW, Chang A, Zhang C, Patterson C, Lee DC (2003) Defective valvulogenesis in HB-EGF and TACE-

null mice is associated with aberrant BMP signaling. *EMBO J* 22:2704–2716.

[36] Krenz M, Yutzey KE, Robbins J (2005) Noonan syndrome mutation Q79R in Shp2 increases proliferation of valve primordia mesenchymal cells via extracellular signal-regulated kinase 1/2 signaling. *Circ Res* 97:813–820.

[37] Alfieri CM, Cheek J, Chakraborty S, Yutzey KE (2010) Wnt signaling in heart valve development and osteogenic gene induction. *Dev Biol* 338:127–135.

[38] Lincoln J, Kist R, Scherer G, Yutzey KE (2007) Sox9 is required for precursor cell expansion and extracellular matrix organization during mouse heart valve development. *Dev Biol* 305:120–132.

[39] Lamers WH, Virágh S, Wessels A, Moorman AF, Anderson RH (1995) Formation of the tricuspid valve in the human heart. *Circulation* 91:111–121.

[40] Lincoln J, Alfieri CM, Yutzey KE (2006) BMP and FGF regulatory pathways control cell lineage diversification of heart valve precursor cells. *Dev Biol* 292:292–302.

[41] Zhao B, Etter L, Hinton RB, Benson DW (2007) BMP and FGF regulatory pathways in semilunar valve precursor cells. *Dev Dyn Off Publ Am Assoc Anat* 236:971–980.

[42] Aikawa E, Whittaker P, Farber M, Mendelson K, Padera RF, Aikawa M, Schoen FJ (2006) Human semilunar cardiac valve remodeling by activated cells from fetus to adult: implications for postnatal adaptation, pathology, and tissue engineering. *Circulation* 113:1344–1352.

[43] Hinton RB, Lincoln J, Deutsch GH, Osinska H, Manning PB, Benson DW, Yutzey KE (2006) Extracellular matrix remodeling and organization in developing and diseased aortic valves. *Circ Res* 98:1431–1438.

[44] Peacock JD, Lu Y, Koch M, Kadler KE, Lincoln J (2008) Temporal and spatial expression of collagens during murine atrioventricular heart valve development and maintenance. *Dev Dyn Off Publ Am Assoc Anat* 237:3051–3058.

[45] Stephens EH, Post AD, Laucirica DR, Grande-Allen KJ (2010) Perinatal changes in mitral and aortic valve structure and composition. *Pediatr Dev Pathol Off J Soc Pediatr Pathol Paediatr Pathol Soc* 13:447–458.

[46] Combs MD, Yutzey KE (2009) Heart valve development: regulatory networks in development and disease. *Circ Res* 105:408–421.

[47] Norris RA, Moreno-Rodriguez RA, Sugi Y, Hoffman S, Amos J, Hart MM, Potts JD, Goodwin RL, Markwald RR (2008) Periostin regulates atrioventricular valve maturation. *Dev Bio*l 316:200–213.

[48] Snider P, Hinton RB, Moreno-Rodriguez RA, et al. (2008) Periostin is required for maturation and extracellular matrix stabilization of noncardiomyocyte lineages of the heart. *Circ Res* 102:752–760.

[49] Rabkin E, Aikawa M, Stone JR, Fukumoto Y, Libby P, Schoen FJ (2001) Activated interstitial myofibroblasts express catabolic enzymes and mediate matrix remodeling in myxomatous heart valves. *Circulation* 104:2525–2532.

[50] Gupta V, Barzilla JE, Mendez JS, Stephens EH, Lee EL, Collard CD, Laucirica R, Weigel PH, Grande-Allen KJ (2009) Abundance and location of proteoglycans and hyaluronan within normal and myxomatous mitral valves. *Cardiovasc Pathol Off J Soc Cardiovasc Pathol* 18:191–197.

[51] Wirrig EE, Hinton RB, Yutzey KE (2011) Differential expression of cartilage and bone-related proteins in pediatric and adult diseased aortic valves. *J Mol Cell Cardiol* 50:561–569.

[52] Cheek JD, Wirrig EE, Alfieri CM, James JF, Yutzey KE (2012) Differential activation of valvulogenic, chondrogenic, and osteogenic pathways in mouse models of myxomatous and calcific aortic valve disease. *J Mol Cell Cardiol* 52:689–700.

[53] Victor S, Nayak VM (1994) The tricuspid valve is bicuspid. *J Heart Valve Dis* 3:27–36.

[54] Anderson RH, Wilcox BR (1995) Understanding cardiac anatomy: the prerequisite for optimal cardiac surgery. *Ann Thorac Surg* 59:1366–1375.

[55] Taramasso M, Vanermen H, Maisano F, Guidotti A, La Canna G, Alfieri O (2012) The growing clinical importance of secondary tricuspid regurgitation. *J Am Coll Cardiol* 59:703–710.

[56] Seccombe JF, Cahill DR, Edwards WD (1993) Quantitative morphology of the normal human tricuspid valve: autopsy study of 24 cases. *Clin Anat Off J Am Assoc Clin Anat Br Assoc Clin Anat* 6:203–212.

[57] Silver M, Lam J, Ranganathan N, Wigle E (1971) Morphology of the human tricuspid valve. *Circulation* 43:333–348.

[58] Sutton III JP, Ho SY, Anderson RH (1995) The forgotten interleaflet triangles: a review of the surgical anatomy of the aortic valve. *Ann Thorac Surg* 59:419–427.

[59] Dreyfus GD, Martin RP, Chan KJ, Dulguerov F, Alexandrescu C (2015) Functional tricuspid regurgitation: a need to revise our understanding. *J Am Coll Cardiol* 65:2331–2336.

[60] Huttin O, Voilliot D, Mandry D, Venner C, Juillière Y, Selton-Suty C (2016) All you need to know about the tricuspid valve: tricuspid valve imaging and tricuspid regurgitation analysis. *Arch Cardiovasc Dis* 109:67–80.

[61] Tretter JT, Sarwark AE, Anderson RH, Spicer DE (2016) Assessment of the anatomical variation to be found in the normal tricuspid valve. *Clin Anat* 29:399–407.

[62] McCarthy KP, Robertus JL, Ho SY (2018) Anatomy and Pathology of the Tricuspid Valve. In: Pract. Man. *Tricuspid Valve Dis*. Springer, pp 3–21.

[63] Paraskevas G, Koutsouflianiotis K, Iliou K (2017) The first descriptions of various anatomical structures and embryological remnants of the heart: A systematic overview. *Int J Cardiol* 227:674–690.

[64] Najib MQ, Vinales KL, Vittala SS, Challa S, Lee HR, Chaliki HP (2012) Predictors for the development of severe tricuspid regurgitation with anatomically normal valve in patients with atrial fibrillation. *Echocardiography* 29:140–146.

[65] Fukuda S, Saracino G, Matsumura Y, Daimon M, Tran H, Greenberg NL, Hozumi T, Yoshikawa J, Thomas JD, Shiota T (2006) Three-dimensional geometry of the tricuspid annulus in healthy subjects and in patients with functional tricuspid regurgitation: a real-time, 3-dimensional echocardiographic study. *Circulation* 114:I–492.

[66] Said SM, Burkhart HM, Schaff HV, Johnson JN, Connolly HM, Dearani JA (2014) When should a mechanical tricuspid valve replacement be considered? *J Thorac Cardiovasc Surg* 148:603–608.

In: The Rediscovered Tricuspid Valve ISBN: 978-1-53616-098-7
Editor: Giacomo Bianchi

Chapter 3

THE DISEASED TRICUSPID VALVE: EPIDEMIOLOGY AND CLINICAL APPROACH TO THE TRICUSPID VALVE DISEASE

Chiara Borrelli*[1,2,*], *MD, Alessandra Burini*[1], *MD, Enrica Manzato*[1], *MD, Cristina Zucchinetti*[1] *MD, and Claudio Passino*[1,3], *MD, PhD
[1]Scuola Superiore Sant'Anna, Pisa, Italy
[2]Division of Emergency Medicine, University of Pisa, Pisa, Italy
[3]Division of Cardiology and Cardiovascular Medicine, Fondazione Toscana "Gabriele Monasterio", Pisa, Italy

ABSTRACT

The recognition of a tricuspid valve disease is often an incidental occurrence during a visit for other reasons. It is often masked by the most prominent symptoms of a left valve disease. Clinically, we recognize two distinct nosological entities, tricuspidal insufficiency, with a higher incidence, and stenosis of the tricuspid valve, which to date has

---

[*] Corresponding Author's E-mail: chiara.borrelli1993@gmail.com.

undergone a radical change in its epidemiology. It is essential, to prepare for the therapy, the knowledge of the epidemiology and the clinical framework of the tricuspid disease.

Keywords: epidemiology, tricuspid valve, tricuspid regurgitation, tricuspid stenosis

INTRODUCTION

The purpose of this chapter is to assess the diseases of the tricuspid valve (TV) from an epidemiological, pathophysiological, clinical, and prognostic point of view.

TV disease is usually neglected in clinical practice, as its diagnosis is generally difficult because symptoms are generally masked by those of left heart disease. However, given the important prognostic impact of TV, as well as an increased interest coming from the developing percutaneous strategies for its repair, it is advisable to revise the main causes of TV disease as well as its clinical manifestations.

This chapter is articulated into two main sections: first, tricuspid stenosis (TS) will be described, followed by tricuspid regurgitation (TR). In each paragraph the epidemiological, etiologic and pathophysiologic aspects of the disease will be analyzed, as well as clinical and prognostic implications.

In particular, for what concerns TR, both primary and secondary causes will be addressed.

Furthermore, key diagnostic aspects of TV disease will be briefly discussed. Finally, clinical conditions in which suspecting TV disease is crucial will be also analysed.

TRICUSPID STENOSIS

Epidemiology

TS is a pathological condition resulting from structural alterations of TV leaflets that obstruct right atrial emptying into the right ventricle (RV) [1].

The epidemiology of TS has changed radically during the past century, ranging from 22 - 44% in the first necroscopic studies of the 1950s to the 1% - 4.4% of the current century [2, 3].

The disparity of those data can be explained with variations in diagnostic criteria (either clinical, echocardiographic and autopsy-based). However, changes in epidemiology of RHD have also played a determinant role [4, 5]. In fact, TS prevalence is lower in industrialized countries (TS, in fact, accounts for 2.4% of all organic TV disease, with an overall prevalence of less than 1%) [3], while it reaches values of 4.4% in countries where antibiotic profilaxis for rheumatic endocarditis is not available [5].

Regarding the congenital form, the incidence is less than 1% and it is considered rare; in these cases, the disease has a slightly higher male predominance [5], while in general TS is more common in elderly women (age > 65 years old) [1, 3].

Etiology

TS can be either congenital or acquired. Among congenital forms, Ebstein anomaly is the most common one; it consists in the apical displacement of the septal tricuspid leaflet with leaflet dysplasia; therefore, only a small portion of the RV remains functional. Mainly, Ebstein abnormality results in TR, but TS is also possible [5].

Among the acquired forms RHD, amyloidosis, carcinoid syndrome, drug-induced toxicity, systemic lupus erythematosus (SLE) or large endocarditis vegetations, and electronic devices (e.g., pacemaker leads) are the most common causes.

Acute rheumatic fever is a latent autoimmune reaction to infections of group A β-hemolytic Streptococci that causes inflammation and fibrosis of valvular tissue, resulting in both mitral and tricuspid stenosis [6]. In some very unusual cases, RHD could be mimicked by cardiac amyloidosis, leading to TS [7].

Carcinoid tumors are neuroendocrine tumors that release high quantities of vasoactive amines, like serotonin, whose metabolites activate pathways of fibroblast proliferation and mitogenesis, leading to valvular fibrosis and stenosis [8]. Similar pro-fibrotic pathways are also activated by some drugs like alkaloid methysergide, fenfluramide and cabergoline [8–10]. SLE causes cardiac involvement in nearly half of patients: valves are involved in as many as 40% of the cases, with less frequency for the TV than for the left-sided valves [11, 12]. TS secondary to aseptic endocarditis has also been reported in Behcet's disease [13].

Tumors very rarely induce valvular stenosis as they have to reach great dimension to extend from the right atrium (RA) to the RV [14]. Nowadays, the most important etiologic factor for TS is pace-maker implantation: endocardial leads passing through its plane are a potential source of damage, rupture and inflammation of the leaflets, a condition often underestimated as it appears many years after device implantation [15]. More rarely, stenosis can be secondary to bacterial endocarditis related to devices implantation [16].

Pathophysiology

The aforementioned different etiologies of TS cause an array of alterations in the valve and surrounding tissue: inflammatory processes lead to fibroblast proliferation that causes leaflet shortening and thickening and, in severe cases, rupture [11, 12, 17]. Moreover, fibrosis can cause fusion of the valvular commissures, as well as thickening and shortening of the chordae tendinae, as seen in RHD [17].

In congenital abnormalities, on the other hand, the leaflets are generally not well developed, the chordae might be shorter or malformed and the annulus is smaller [17]. All these anomalies affect blood passage from the RA to the RV, therefore generating a diastolic pressure gradient, which increases during inspiration (when the blood flow through the valve is greater) and decreases in expiration (when the blood flow is reduced). Given the extremely low pressure in the RA, even a small pressure increase is enough to determine systemic venous congestion, with clinical consequences (Figure 1).

In fact, increased central venous pressure leads to edema formation in the Disse area, with subsequent hepatic fibrosis. Furthermore, increased central venous pressure is also directly mechanically responsible for hepatic damage, accelerating the processes of cirrhosis and liver failure. Finally, increased central venous pressure is responsible for fluid leakage in the third space, with peripheral and generalized edema [18].

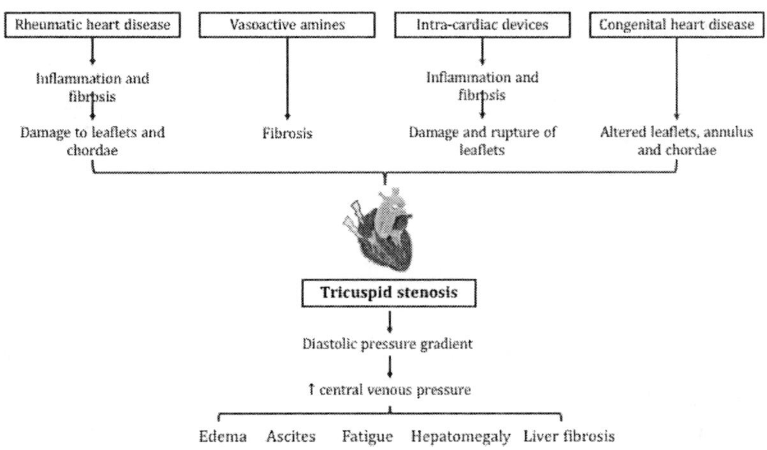

Figure 1. Pathophysiology of tricuspid valve stenosis.

Clinical Manifestations

For the aforementioned reasons, the clinical presentation of TS is dominated by venous congestion and its consequences: hepatomegaly, which can cause abdominal discomfort and pain; peripheral edemas; ascites or, in the most severe cases, anasarca. Moreover, increased central venous pressure related to TS leads to liver fibrosis, cirrhosis and, eventually, liver failure.

Those systemic symptoms are predominant and usually severe, especially when compared to the degree of dyspnea, which usually increases in case of concomitant left heart disease; in addition to that, jugular veins can be distended, even to the point in which the patient complains of a throbbing in the neck. Finally, cardiac blood output is reduced because of reduced blood flow to the left chambers of the heart, leading to fatigue and asthenia [5].

During auscultation, in rare cases of severe TS, it is possible to appreciate a diastolic rumble along the left lower sternal border, which accentuates during inspiration or with other maneuvers that increase blood flow through the valve. Furthermore, with cardiac catheterization, the pressures in the RV, left atrium and pulmonary circulation are normal or only slightly elevated [5, 19].

Finally, electrocardiographic (EKG) findings generally include sinus rhythm; however, in severe TS with RA enlargement and hypertrophy, a P pulmonale might be detected.

Prognosis

The prognosis of TS greatly depends on its etiology, with an overall mortality rate around 5%. Mild to moderate TS is asymptomatic and doesn't require treatment, whereas severe TS must be surgically corrected, with a relevant perioperative mortality, ranging between 9 - 20% [20].

Long-term survival after TV replacement is variable and depends upon the etiology [20, 21]. However, in severe TS timing of the surgical operation is essential, as progression to end-stage heart failure still remains the first cause of death in those patients, coupled with liver disease and stroke [22, 23].

Furthermore, other factors affecting morbidity and mortality in TS patients include: pulmonary hypertension and dyspnea [22].

Currently, percutaneous approaches alternative to classic surgery are being studied, even though long-term results and prognostic efficacy are still unknown [24]. However, due to the rarity of the disease, specific prognostic studies are difficult to obtain. Therefore, prognostic factors in TS are poorly described and further studies are needed to better characterize this condition.

Tricuspid Regurgitation

Epidemiology

TR is a pathological condition in which blood backflows from the RV to the RA because of an incompetency of the valve.

Among right sided valvuopathies, TR is extremely more common than TS [25]. TR can be distinguished in primary TR, generally caused by a structural valvular defect (which accounts for around 10% of the cases), and secondary TR, which is generally caused by tricuspid annular dilatation due to geometric alterations of the RV with or without concomitant left heart disease [1, 26].

More solid data on TR epidemiology came with the Framingham Heart Study, that described a prevalence of 82% in men and 85.7% in women [25]. TR severity increases with age. Interestingly, TR is more prevalent in young women while it has a male predominance in the elderly (moderate TR in men and women < 40 years old: 0% and 1.2%, respectively, moderate TR in men and women > 70 years old: 25.8% and 5.6%, respectively) [1].

Degenerative etiologies of TR are more prevalent in developed countries, whereas endocarditis and RHD are more common in the developing countries and among intravenous drug users, as explained in the following paragraph [3, 19].

Etiology

TR can be categorized as congenital or acquired, and primary or secondary depending on whether or not it is related to other cardiac diseases such as mitral valve disease (also called functional TR) [27].

For what concerns primary congenital TR, it is more commonly related to Ebstein anomaly, as explained before [5].

Acquired primary TR, on the other hand, can be related to several diseases. RHD, myxoma, sarcoidosis, SLE, pace-maker leads, carcinoid or drug abuse are principal causes of acquired primary TR, as they primarily damage TV leaflets [12].

Bacterial endocarditis generally affects patients with a history of alcohol or drug abuse, neoplasms, infected indwelling catheters, extensive burns and immunodeficiency and it is a potential cause of leaflets destruction and perforation, chordal rupture, valve restriction and, eventually, TR [3, 12].

Endocardial fibroelastosis and endomyocardial biopsies, on the other hand, primarily cause damage both to the chordae and the papillary muscles [28]. Connective tissue disorders (mainly Marfan and Ehlers Danlos syndromes) can also cause TR, generally due to a floppy valve with concomitant annulus dilatation [5].

Carcinoid syndrome or drugs that act on serotonergic pathways can also lead to poor leaflet coaptation due to increased production of serotonin and its metabolites, as explained in the paragraph 2.2 [8, 10, 29]. Renal tumors invading the inferior vena cava and reaching the RA, as well as atrial myxomas or large aneurysms of the sinus of Valsalva also determine TR by partially obstructing blood flow and distorting the tricuspid annulus, causing intra-annular or peri-annular impingement [12].

Blunt trauma is another important cause of primary acquired TR: rapid elevation of RV pressure, in fact, is responsible for leaflet damage, papillary muscle damage or chordal rupture [30, 31]. Finally, atrial fibrillation accounts for 85% of the cases of primary acquired TR (due to systole-related stress) mainly because of progressive distortion of the annulus, as explained in the following paragraph.

However, TR can be also secondary to atrial fibrillation-induced RV failure, as explained in the following paragraph [12, 32].

Finally, permanent pacing and implantable cardioverter defibrillators can accelerate TR progression, as the inserted catheters determine leaflet fibrosis and displacement and, in severe cases, rupture (as explained in the paragraph 2.2) [33, 34].

Secondary TR, also called functional TR (FTR), on the other hand, represents 85 - 90% of TR and it is related to left or right heart disease, annular dilatation and subsequent reduced leaflet coaptation [26].

For what concerns left heart disease, FTR can be found in 30 - 50% of patients with mitral regurgitation (MR), but it can also be described in mitral and aortic stenosis, as those are all conditions that lead to pulmonary hypertension (PH) [35].

Indeed, PH is a crucial etiologic factor of FTR: in an echocardiographic study of 242 patients with severe TR, 72% presented significant PH (defined as pulmonary artery pressure > 50 mmHg) [36]. Interestingly, TR can be described in up to 77% of patients with PH due to chronic obstructive pulmonary disease, therefore underlining the pathophysiologic interdependence between increased workload of the right heart and TR [37].

Finally, TR can be described in patients with RV remodeling and annular dilatation due to RV dysfunction as in RV infarction, amyloidosis, acromegaly or pulmonary valve disease, as explained in the following paragraph [5, 38].

Pathophysiology

In TR, different etiologic backgrounds can lead to either pure TR or concomitant TR and TS.

In pure TR, there is usually leaflet thickening and annular dilatation, while in concomitant stenosis there is also commissural fusion and chordal thickening [17].

In either case, central venous pressure increases and cardiac output decreases because of both reduced RV stroke volume and reduced LV function secondary to RV alterations (Figure 2). Therefore, the RV progressively enlarges further progressing TR [26, 38].

In primary TR, the valvular apparatus is either abnormal or primary attacked with leaflet and chordal damage, as mentioned above. In particular, in Ebstein's abnormality, the leaflets are enlarged and abnormally inserted and the annular circumference is increased [39].

Endomyocardial fibrosis and RHD primarily cause shortening of the chordae tendinae with fibrosis and valvular thickening, while myxedema can determine valve prolapse, valve thickening, chordae elongation and annulus dilatation [5, 12, 27].

Carcinoid disease, on the other hand, determines the formation of plaques both on the ventricular side of leaflets and on the ventricular wall, which tend to adhere to each other and block proper coaptation [39].

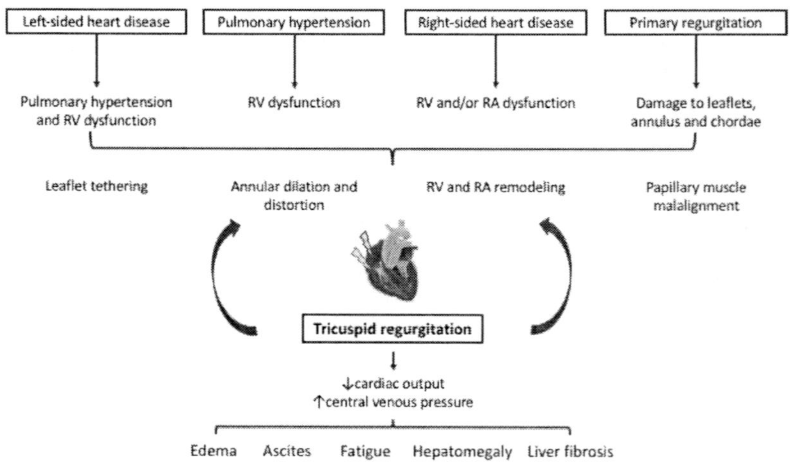

Figure 2. Pathophysiology of tricuspid regurgitation.

Finally, pacemaker leads and defibrillators can alter valve physiology promoting leaflet distortion and preventing proper coaptation, leading to inflammation and fibrosis and, in severe cases, leaflet perforation [33, 34]. As a result of the primary process affecting the TV, right heart volume increases and the annulus progressively dilates, worsening the phenomenon [40, 41].

In FTR, on the other hand, the TV is not directly affected but pressure and/or volume overload on the RV (and, more rarely, on the RA) are the primary pathophysiological determinants. In particular, left heart disease, PH and right heart disease are the key determinants of RV pressure/volume overload.

In left-sided heart disease (mainly MR), increased pressure in the left heart leads to PH and FTR, as further explained below [41]. However, LV dysfunction and LA enlargement were found to be associated with moderate and severe TR independently of the degree of PH [36]. This finding is thought to be related to the functional interdependence of the LV and the RV, that share muscular fibers as well as the septum and a biochemical milieu [42]. Indeed, 20 - 40% of the RV systolic pressure and volume output come from LV contraction [38]; therefore, a decrease in LV function also decreases RV output contributing to TR development [41]. Furthermore, LV remodeling alters the interventricular septum, where the TV septal leaflet and papillary muscles are attached, further progressing TR [36, 43].

PH both due to left-sided heart disease or primary pulmonary disease arguably remains the most common and important determinant of TR. In fact, PH increases pressures on the right heart, leading to RV enlargement and functional impairment with annular dilatation and leaflet tethering [38, 44, 45]. According to some authors, leaflet tethering is the main mechanism for TR in PH, as the RV dilates in length but not in its basal diameters, leading to papillary muscles displacement (and therefore leaflet tethering) rather than extreme annular dilatation [46]. Interestingly, not all patients with PH develop TR, suggesting that other mechanisms beyond pressure overload, such as RA enlargement or TV annular dilatation might play a role [36].

Finally, TR can also be determined by diseases affecting directly the right heart, such as pulmonary valve (PV) disease or atrial fibrillation. In case of PV disease, there can either be a pressure (PV stenosis) or a volume overload (PV regurgitation); both of these lead to RV enlargement and progressive dysfunction [5, 38]. In case of atrial fibrillation, instead, there is no pressure or volume overload, but rather a RA dysfunction damaging the valve. Indeed, case-control studies have suggested that atrial fibrillation progressively induces RA dilatation, which worsens with time; RA volume is in turn strongly correlated to the annular diameter of TV; therefore, RA dilation results in annulus dilatation and subsequent leaflet mal-coaptation with TR development [47]. In addition, atrial fibrillation can determine loss of contraction of the myocardium surrounding the annulus, which can also lead to TR [26]. However, TR itself can promote RA enlargement and, therefore, atrial fibrillation, thus promoting the vicious circle [42, 47].

Clinical Manifestations

TR, even when significant, is often asymptomatic; moreover, given the often-combined existence of TR and LV disease, symptoms of TR might be masked. However, when PH develops, the patient is more markedly symptomatic [5].

Both symptoms of left and right heart disease can be appreciated: left heart pathology as well as impaired filling leads to asthenia, fatigue, hypotension and pulmonary congestion; right ventricular disease, on the other hand, leads to venous and hepatic congestion, with ascites, peripheral edema, increased jugular pressure and, in severe cases, anasarca or cachexia. As mentioned before, it is possible to notice those signs and symptoms simultaneously [42]. Pitting peripheral edema is common in patients with severe TR, as well as hepatic congestion and hepatomegaly. Ascites can also be found when performing a physical examination. In addition to that, jugular veins might appear as pulsatile and distended; systolic eyeball pulsations have also been described [5].

In case of severe and prolonged TR, signs of liver failure (such as jaundice) can be appreciated, as well as peripheral cyanosis, hypotension and, ultimately, cardiac cachexia [5]. During auscultation it is possible to appreciate a soft systolic murmur at the lower left sternal border, which is increased by inspiration [46], hepatic compression or leg raising [5, 19]; this murmur is initially pan-systolic but it can become proto-systolic and of lower intensity with disease progression, because of reduced pressure gradient between RV and RA [19]. In addition, a third heart sound coming from the RV and accentuated by inspiration can also be appreciated [5].

When PH is present, the second heart sound is accentuated and TV murmur can be best appreciated in the parasternal or, occasionally, sub-xiphoid region.

Auscultation of the jugular veins can reveal a systolic thrill and a murmur, and measurement of central venous pressure with invasive cardiac catheterism shows a prominent systolic wave, whose decent is sharp [5]. Similar to TS, in sinus rhythm on EKG a prominent P wave might be described; however, atrial fibrillation and flutter are also common EKG findings.

Prognosis

The prognosis of TR is strictly related to the severity of the disease. More specifically, in a study on 5,223 patients with TR, one-year survival was 91.7% with no TR, 90.3% with mild TR, 78.9% with moderate TR and 63.9% with severe TR [48]. At 3 years follow up, the survival rate of moderate or severe TR is around 40% [49]. Moderate or severe TR (both primary and secondary) is an independent risk factor for mortality and it is associated with poor outcome regardless of LV ejection fraction, RV dilation, RV and LV dysfunction, inferior vena cava dilation and age [48].

When TR coexists with PH, it can easily lead to heart failure negatively affecting prognosis [5]. However, recent studies have demonstrated that even patients with isolated TR present an excess mortality of 3.8% per year [50].

Nonetheless, recent studies have underlined how RV dysfunction greatly impacts on TR prognosis [51]. Those data are of particular interest when related to surgical approaches to TR. In fact, TR surgery is usually delayed due to lack of solid prognostic data as well as information regarding the correct timing for surgery, therefore leading to progressive RV dysfunction that might have an impact on prognosis [24].

From a surgical standpoint, TV repair is usually preferred over TV replacement, as it is associated with less complications; however, there is no significant difference in early mortality (3.4% and 3.1% respectively), nor in survival at 10 years from intervention (70% and 72%) [52, 53].

Operative mortality of TV surgery ranges between 2% and 25%, depending on hospital expertise as well as on comorbidities, RA pressure and RV dysfunction, stressing again that an early intervention could ameliorate the outcome [50, 53].

Significant risk factors for overall mortality are age and preoperative left ventricle dysfunction, hemoglobin < 10 g/dL and intravenous inotrope use [52]. However, data on long-term outcomes of TR surgery are lacking [53]. Up to 20% of the patients present recurrent severe TR 5 years after intervention, but reoperation is not often performed, as it is associated with high perioperative mortality (around 37%) [50].

At the moment, different percutaneous TV interventions are under development, but clinical experience is still limited and very few prognostic data are available and, even though the first results are promising, there is still need for larger studies [53].

Clinical Approach to Tricuspid Valve Disease

When diagnosed, TV disease can be better qualified with different imaging techniques. The first and most important one is cardiac ultrasound, but also cardiac computed tomography (CT) can provide additional information while cardiac magnetic resonance imaging (MRI) is nowadays the gold standard [54]. Finally, EKG and chest X-ray can also provide the physician with additional useful information.

Echocardiography is the most important imaging modality to identify the etiology, assess the geometry and function of the valve and the right heart chambers, determine the severity of valve disease, and evaluate pulmonary artery pressure, which can help in deciding whether TR is primary or secondary [5, 24, 26]. Transthoracic echocardiography is the first choice and it is usually done in two dimensions, but can also be done in three, which allows simultaneous observation of all three leaflets and their commissures [5]. Transesophageal echocardiography, on the other hand, provides with important information during TV surgery and it is becoming the imaging modality of choice for the new percutaneous approaches. However, due to the well-known limitations of ultrasound, further diagnostic studies are usually performed. Cardiac MRI provides with very accurate information for both a morphological and a functional evaluation of the TV and heart chambers [26]. However, it is not always available, it is expensive and is often contraindicated by the presence of device leads or other metallic implants [54].

Multi-slice CT, on the other hand, has a great spatial resolution and can therefore offer very detailed anatomical information [55].

Finally, EKG and chest X-ray can also arise clinical suspicion or give additional information. This exam will frequently show atrial fibrillation – as a result of right atrial enlargement – and right bundle branch block, which however are not specific to TR; in case of severe RA enlargement, a *P pulmonale* can also be present. X-ray scans shows cardiomegaly with a prominent inferior right arch, suggesting RA enlargement; it is also possible to detect signs of hemodynamic overload such as a dilated azygos vein, pleural diffusion and diaphragm elevation due to ascites [5, 42].

Conclusion: When to Suspect Tricuspid Valve Disease

Since even severe TV disease is often asymptomatic, oftentimes the diagnosis is made during a routine examination for other symptoms, predominantly left-heart disease symptoms [26, 40]. From a clinical standpoint, TV disease is generally diagnosed during a routine clinical ultrasound. However, suspecting and assessing TV disease is crucial from both a therapeutic and prognostic point of view.

TS should be considered always in presence of left sided valvulopathies in patients with a history of Streptococcal infection or carcinoid disease.

TR, on the other hand, should always be suspected in patients with left sided heart disease such as MR or heart failure.

RV function and TV function should always be assessed in patients with pulmonary diseases such ah PH or chronic obstructive pulmonary disease, in which increased workload on the right chambers of the heart might negatively impact on their function. Finally, TV should always be assessed in patients with a disorder of cardiac rhythm such as atrial fibrillation or flutter.

Clinically, direct symptoms of TV disease are usually subtle and often masked by symptoms of left heart disease. In clinical practice, patients often complain of dyspnea secondary to heart failure and or MR, resulting in pleural effusion and therefore increased difficulty breathing. Rarely, TV disease (mainly TR) can be suspected with the appreciation on physical examination of a soft systolic murmur at the left sternal border that changes in intensity with inspiration [46].

Patients presenting with symptoms of right sided failure (hepatomegaly, ascites, peripheral edema) without dyspnea or signs and symptoms of hypoperfusion should always be worked up in the suspicion of primary TR or TR secondary to RV failure. Finally, patients presenting with abdominal discomfort, hepatomegaly and ascites in absence of signs of primitive hepatic disease should also be evaluated from a cardiac standpoint, and a cardiac cirrhosis should promptly be assessed.

References

[1] Supino, P. G., Borer, J. S., Preibisz, J. & Bornstein, A. (2006). The Epidemiology of Valvular Heart Disease: a Growing Public Health Problem. *Heart Fail Clin*, *2*, 379–393.

[2] Kitchin, A. & Turner, R. (1964). Diagnosis and treatment of tricuspid stenosis. *Brit Heart J*, *26*.

[3] Iung, B. & Vahanian, A. (2011). Epidemiology of acquired valvular heart disease. *Can J Cardiol*. doi: 10.1016/j.cjca.2014.03.022.

[4] Duval, X., Delahaye, F., Alla, F., et al. (2012). Temporal trends in infective endocarditis in the context of prophylaxis guideline modifications: Three successive population-based surveys. *J Am Coll Cardiol*, *59*, 1968–1976.

[5] Mann, D. L., Zipes, D. P., Libby, P., Bonow, R. O. & Braunwald, E. (2015). *Braunwald's heart disease: A textbook of cardiovascular medicine, Tenth*. doi: 10.1016/B978-1-4377-0398-6.00043-3.

[6] Tibazarwa, K. B., Volmink, J. A. & Mayosi, B. M. (2008). Incidence of acute rheumatic fever in the world: A systematic review of population-based studies. *Heart*, *94*, 1534–1540.

[7] Kim, K. H., Park, C. H., Park, H. S., Kim, Y. R. & Choi, E. Y. (2014). Amyloidosis-induced tricuspid stenosis mimicking rheumatic heart disease. *Eur Heart J Cardiovasc Imaging*, *15*, 1167.

[8] Zanettini, R., Antonini, A., Gatto, G., Gentile, R., Tesei, S. & Pezzoli, G. (2007). Valvular Heart Disease and the Use of Dopamine Agonists for Parkinson's Disease. *N Engl J Med*. doi: 10.1056/NEJMoa054830.

[9] Mast, S. T., Jollis, J. G., Ryan, T., Anstrom, K. J. & Crary, J. L. (2001). The progression of fenfluramine-associated valvular heart disease assessed by echocardiography. *Ann Intern Med*, *134*, 261–266.

[10] Seghatol, F. F. & Rigolin, V. H. (2002). Appetite suppressants and valvular heart disease. *Curr Opin Cardiol*. doi: 10.1097/00001573-200209000-00007.

[11] Moyssakis, I., Tektonidou, M. G., Vasilliou, V. A., Samarkos, M., Votteas, V. & Moutsopoulos, H. M. (2007). Libman-Sacks Endocarditis in Systemic Lupus Erythematosus: Prevalence, Associations, and Evolution. *Am J Med*. doi: 10.1016/j.amjmed.2007.01.024.

[12] Adler, D. S. (2017). Non-functional tricuspid valve disease. *Ann Cardiothorac Surg*, *6*, 204–213.

[13] Lee, H. S., Choi, W. S., Kim, K. H., et al. (2011). Aseptic endocarditis in Behçet's disease presenting as tricuspid valve stenosis. *Korean Circ J*, *41*, 399–401.

[14] Taylor, J. E., Harless, A., Shah, L., Sangeeta, Huang., Gilliland, Y. E. & Qamruddin, S. (2018). Large Primary Cardiac Lymphoma causing functional tricuspid valve stenosis. *Tex Heart Inst J*, *45*, 275–276.

[15] Husain, A., Raja, F. T., Fatallah, A., Fadel, B., Alsanei, A., Raja, F. T. & AlGhamdi, B. (2017). Tricuspid stenosis: An emerging disease in cardiac implantable electronic devices era. Case report and literature review. *J Cardiol Cases*, *15*, 190–193.

[16] Nisanci, Y., Yilmaz, E., Oncul, A. & Ozsaruhan, O. (1999). Predominant tricuspid stenosis secondary to bacterial endocarditis in a patient with permanent pacemaker and balloon dilatation of the stenosis. *PACE - Pacing Clin Electrophysiol*, *22*, 393–396.

[17] Waller, B. F., Howard, J. & Fess, S. (1995). Pathology of tricuspid valve stenosis and pure tricuspid regurgitation—Part I. *Clin Cardiol*, *18*, 167–174.

[18] Wong, F. S. (2017). The liver in heart failure. *Handb Liver Dis*, *6*, 293–307.

[19] Coffey, S., Rayner, J., Newton, J. & Prendergast, B. D. (2014). Right-sided valve disease. *Int J Clin Pract*, *68*, 1221–1226.

[20] Scully, H. E. & Armstrong, C. S. (1995). Tricuspid valve replacement: Fifteen years of experience with mechanical prostheses and bioprostheses. *J Thorac Cardiovasc Surg*, *109*, 1035–1041.

[21] Castillo, J. G., Filsoufi, F., Rahmanian, P. B., Anyanwu, A., Zacks, J. S., Warner, R. R. P. & Adams, D. H. (2008). Early and Late Results of Valvular Surgery for Carcinoid Heart Disease. *J Am Coll Cardiol*, *51*, 1507–1509.

[22] Diaof, M., Ba, S. A., Kane, A., Sarr, M., Diop, I. B. & Diouf, S. M. (2004). *Tricuspid valve stenosis. A prospective study of 35 cases*. Dakar Méd.

[23] Filsoufi, F., Anyanwu, A. C., Salzberg, S. P., Frankel, T., Cohn, L. H. & Adams, D. H. (2005). Long-Term Outcomes of Tricuspid Valve Replacement in the Current Era. *Ann Thorac Surg*, *80*, 845–850.

[24] Falk, V., Baumgartner, H., Bax, J. J., et al. (2017). 2017 ESC/EACTS Guidelines for the management of valvular heart disease. *Eur J Cardio-Thorac Surg Off J Eur Assoc Cardio-Thorac Surg*, *52*, 616–664.

[25] Singh, J. P., Evans, J. C., Levy, D., Larson, M. G., Freed, L. A., Fuller, D. L., Lehman, B. & Benjamin, E. J. (1999). Prevalence and clinical determinants of mitral, tricuspid, and aortic regurgitation (The Framingham Heart Study). *Am J Cardiol*, *83*, 897–902.

[26] Mas, P. T., Rodríguez-Palomares, J. F. & Antunes, M. J. (2015). Secondary tricuspid valve regurgitation: A forgotten entity. *Heart*, *101*, 1840–1848.

[27] Mrsic, Z., Hopkins, S. P., Antevil, J. L. & Mullenix, P. S. (2018). Valvular Heart Disease. *Prim Care*, *45*, 81–94.

[28] Nguyen, V., Cantarovich, M., Cecere, R. & Giannetti, N. (2005). Tricuspid regurgitation after cardiac transplantation: how many biopsies are too many? *J Heart Lung Transplant Off Publ Int Soc Heart Transplant*. doi: 10.1016/j.healun.2004.07.007.

[29] Mason, J. W., Billingham, M. E. & Friedman, J. P. (1977). Methysergide-induced heart disease. A case of multivalvular and myocardial fibrosis. *Circulation*. doi: 10.1161/01.CIR.56.5.889.

[30] Dounis, G., Matsakas, E., Poularas, J., Papakonstantinou, K., Kalogeromitros, A. & Karabinis, A. (2002). Traumatic tricuspid insufficiency: A case report with a review of the literature. *Eur J Emerg Med*, *9*, 258–261.

[31] De Biasi, A. R., Seastedt, K. P., Eachempati, S. R. & Salemi, A. (2015). Common Cause of Mortality in Trauma but Manageable Nonetheless. *Circulation*. doi: 10.1161/circulationaha.115. 016061.

[32] Ong, K., Yu, G. & Jue, J. (2014). Prevalence and spectrum of conditions associated with severe tricuspid regurgitation. *Echocardiography*, *31*, 558–562.

[33] Lin, G., Nishimura, R. A., Connolly, H. M., Dearani, J. A., Sundt, T. M. & Hayes, D. L. (2005). Severe symptomatic tricuspid valve regurgitation due to permanent pacemaker or implantable cardioverter-defibrillator leads. *J Am Coll Cardiol*, *45*, 1672–1675.

[34] Kim, J. B., Spevack, D. M., Tunick, P. A., Bullinga, J. R., Kronzon, I., Chinitz, L. A. & Reynolds, H. R. (2008). The Effect of Transvenous Pacemaker and Implantable Cardioverter Defibrillator Lead Placement on Tricuspid Valve Function: An Observational Study. *J Am Soc Echocardiogr*. doi: 10.1016/j.echo.2007.05.022.

[35] Dreyfus, G. D., Corbi, P. J., Chan, K. M. J. & Bahrami, T. (2005). Secondary tricuspid regurgitation or dilatation: which should be the criteria for surgical repair? *Ann Thorac Surg*, *79*, 127–132.

[36] Mutlak, D., Lessick, J., Reisner, S. A., Aronson, D., Dabbah, S. & Agmon, Y. (2007). Echocardiography-based Spectrum of Severe Tricuspid Regurgitation: The Frequency of Apparently Idiopathic Tricuspid Regurgitation. *J Am Soc Echocardiogr*, *20*, 405–408.

[37] Higham, M. A., Dawson, D., Joshi, J., Nihoyannopoulos, P. & Morrell, N. W. (2001). Utility of echocardiography in assessment of pulmonary hypertension secondary to COPD. *Eur Respir J*, *17*, 350–355.

[38] Haddad, F., Doyle, R., Murphy, D. J. & Hunt, S. A. (2008). Right ventricular function in cardiovascular disease, part II: Pathophysiology, clinical importance, and management of right ventricular failure. *Circulation*, *117*, 1717–1731.

[39] Waller, B. F., Howard, J. & Fess, S. (1995). Pathology of tricuspid valve stenosis and pure tricuspid regurgitation—Part II. *Clin Cardiol*, *18*, 167–174.

[40] Arsalan, M., Walther, T., Smith, R. L. & Grayburn, P. A. (2017). Tricuspid regurgitation diagnosis and treatment. *Eur Heart J*, *38*, 634–638.

[41] Antunes, M. J., Rodríguez-Palomares, J., Prendergast, B., et al. (2017). Management of tricuspid valve regurgitation: Position statement of the European Society of Cardiology Working Groups of Cardiovascular Surgery and Valvular Heart Disease. *Eur J Cardiothorac Surg*, *52*, 1022–1030.

[42] Rogers, J. H. & Bolling, S. F. (2009). The tricuspid valve: Current perspective and evolving management of tricuspid regurgitation. *Circulation*, *119*, 2718–2725.

[43] Fukuda, S., Saracino, G., Matsumura, Y., Daimon, M., Tran, H., Greenberg, N. L., Hozumi, T., Yoshikawa, J., Thomas, J. D. & Shiota, T. (2006). Three-dimensional geometry of the tricuspid annulus in healthy subjects and in patients with functional tricuspid regurgitation: a real-time, 3-dimensional echocardiographic study. *Circulation*, *114*, I–492.

[44] Taramasso, M., Vanermen, H., Maisano, F., Guidotti, A., La Canna, G. & Alfieri, O. (2012). The growing clinical importance of secondary tricuspid regurgitation. *J Am Coll Cardiol*, *59*, 703–710.

[45] Medvedofsky, D., Aronson, D., Gomberg-Maitland, M., Thomeas, V., Rich, S., Spencer, K., Mor-Avi, V., Addetia, K., Lang, R. M. & Shiran, A. (2017). Tricuspid regurgitation progression and regression in pulmonary arterial hypertension: Implications for right ventricular and tricuspid valve apparatus geometry and patients outcome. *Eur Heart J Cardiovasc Imaging*, *18*, 86–94.

[46] Topilsky, Y., Khanna, A., Le Toumeau, T., Park, S., Michelena, H., Suri, R., Mahoney, D. W., Enriquez-Sarano, M. (2012). Clinical context and mechanism of functional tricuspid regurgitation in patients with and without pulmonary hypertension. *Circ Cardiovasc Imaging*, *5*, 314–323.

[47] Najib, M. Q., Vinales, K. L., Vittala, S. S., Challa, S., Lee, H. R. & Chaliki, H. P. (2012). Predictors for the development of severe tricuspid regurgitation with anatomically normal valve in patients with atrial fibrillation. *Echocardiography*, *29*, 140–146.

[48] Nath, J., Foster, E. & Heidenreich, P. A. (2004). Impact of tricuspid regurgitation on long-term survival. *J Am Coll Cardiol*, *43*, 405–409.

[49] Lange, R., Piazza, N. & Günther, T. (2017). Tricuspid valve regurgitation: Indications and operative techniques. *Herz*, *42*, 653–661.

[50] Fender, E. A., Zack, C. J. & Nishimura, R. A. (2018). Isolated tricuspid regurgitation: Outcomes and therapeutic interventions. *Heart*, *104*, 798–806.

[51] Dietz, M. F., Prihadi, E. A., Van Der Bijl, P., Goedemans, L., Gursoy, E., Van Genderen, O. S., Ajmone Marsan, N., Delgado, V.

& Bax, J. J. (2018). Prognostic implications of staging significant tricuspid regurgitation: new paradigm for risk stratification. *Eur Heart J*. doi: 10.1093/eurheartj/ehy566.5320.

[52] Chang, H. W., Jeong, D. S., Cho, Y. H., Sung, K., Kim, W. S., Lee, Y. T. & Park, P. W. (2017). Tricuspid Valve Replacement vs. Repair in Severe Tricuspid Regurgitation. *Circ J*, *81*, 330–338.

[53] Al-Hijji, M., Fender, E. A., El Sabbagh, A. & Holmes, D. R. (2017). Current Treatment Strategies for Tricuspid Regurgitation. *Curr Cardiol Rep*, *19*, 9–11.

[54] Rodés-Cabau, J., Taramasso, M. & O'Gara, P. T. (2016). Diagnosis and treatment of tricuspid valve disease: current and future perspectives. *The Lancet*, *388*, 2431–2442.

[55] Vogel-Claussen, J., Pannu, H., Spevak, P. J., Fishman, E. K. & Bluemke, D. A. (2006). Cardiac valve assessment with MR imaging and 64-section multi-detector row CT. *Radiogr Rev Publ Radiol Soc N Am Inc*, *26*, 1769–84.

In: The Rediscovered Tricuspid Valve ISBN: 978-1-53616-098-7
Editor: Giacomo Bianchi

Chapter 4

NON-INVASIVE IMAGING OF THE TRICUSPID VALVE – ULTRASOUNDS: TRANSTHORACIC AND TRANSESOPHAGEAL ECHOCARDIOGRAPHY

Giulia Elena Mandoli*[1]*, MD
Alberto Giannoni*[2,3,*]*, MD, PhD, Chiara Borrelli*[2,4]*, MD
and Matteo Cameli*[1]*, MD, PhD
[1]Department of Cardiovascular Disease,
University of Siena, Siena, Italy
[2]Scuola Superiore Sant'Anna, Pisa, Italy
[3]Division of Cardiology and Cardiovascular Medicine –
Fondazione Toscana "G. Monasterio," Pisa, Italy
[4]Division of Emergency Medicine, University of Pisa, Pisa, Italy

* Corresponding Author's E-mail: alberto.giannoni@ftgm.it.

ABSTRACT

The evaluation and quantification of the tricuspid pathology is in most cases entrusted to ultrasound: through transthoracic and transesophageal doppler echocardiogram it is possible to obtain all the information necessary to establish morphology, degree and extent of the pathology of the tricuspid valve, placing it in the hemodynamic context in vivo and especially being able to assess it entirely with the right ventricle and the concomitant left-sided heart disease.

Keywords: tricuspid valve, ultrasound, assessment, follow-up

INTRODUCTION

An accurate medical history and physical examination of the patient suffering from tricuspid valve (TV) disease must necessarily be followed by non-invasive ultrasound imaging. Echocardiography remains the cornerstone of the diagnosis of diseases of the right heart and in particular of the tricuspid valve. The purpose of the examination is not only to confirm or not the presence of a valve regurgitation or stenosis, but also to provide detailed anatomical elements that can guide the clinician towards the etiology and the most appropriate treatment, both pharmacological and/or structural. The use of continuous doppler (CW) is useful to derive the mean gradient in tricuspid stenosis, while a combined use of CW and color flow Doppler allows the quantification of the degree of regurgitation. Moreover, the determination of the etiology requires the careful evaluation of the leaflets and their morphology, of the annulus dimensions, of the subvalvular apparatus and also of the right ventricle.

TRANS-THORACIC ECHOCARDIOGRAPHY OF THE TRICUSPID VALVE

Anatomic Assessment of the Tricuspid Valve

Transthoracic echocardiography (TTE) is the first and most used approach for this purpose thanks to its non-invasiveness, low costs and to the possibility of repeated bed-side examinations.

The TV is the most apical heart valve and also the largest, with an annular area of about 8–12 cm^2 [1]. As for mitral valve, it is more correct to describe a TV apparatus, composed of annulus, leaflets, chordae tendineae, papillary muscles and myocardium of both right atrium and right ventricle. The annulus is ovoid and larger, along its mediolateral plane, than longer in about 30% of patients [2]. It has a three-dimensional (3D) saddle shape in which the antero-lateral and posterior-septal segments are the closest to right ventricular (RV) apex while the antero-septal and posterolateral portions to the right atrium.

The described typical anatomic property is lost in case of TV disease. Tricuspid annulus (TA) diameter has different cut-off values according to the site of measurement and to the time point during cardiac cycle, varying between 25 and 39 mm [3], being the annular fractional systo-diastolic shortening about 25% [4]. Actually, the cycle cut-point and the best two-dimensional TTE view in which the annulus should be assessed are still quite controversial.

By the way, the European Society of Cardiology (ESC) 2017 guidelines for the management of valvular heart disease define TA dilatation as ≥40 mm or >21 mm/m^2 [5]. As we have seen in chapter 2, the tricuspid valve has three leaflets, namely the anterior leaflet (also called upper, infundibular or lateral), the posterior leaflet (also called lower, dorsal or mural) and the septal leaflet. The anterior is the largest one, the posterior leaflet has different scallops, the septal one is the smallest and the most apical. Subvalvular apparatus is made of three papillary muscles, anterior, posterior and septal, that attach to the leaflets, usually more than one, via true chordae tendineae. However, there is an extreme anatomical variability of these structures.

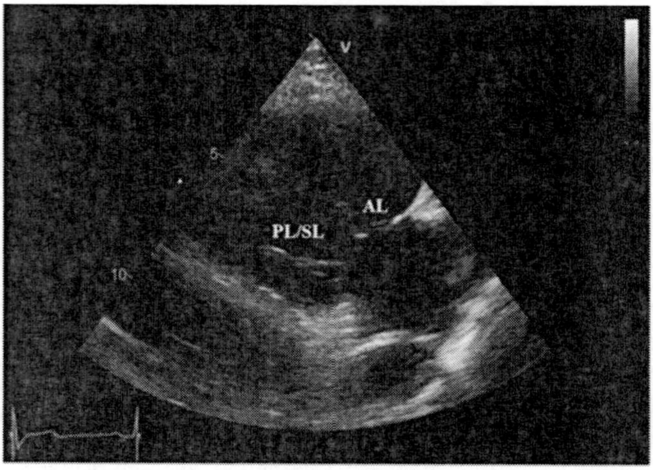

Figure 1A. Two-dimensional transthoracic echocardiography: parasternal right ventricular inflow long axis view. It is obtained by a downward tilting of the probe from a conventional parasternal.

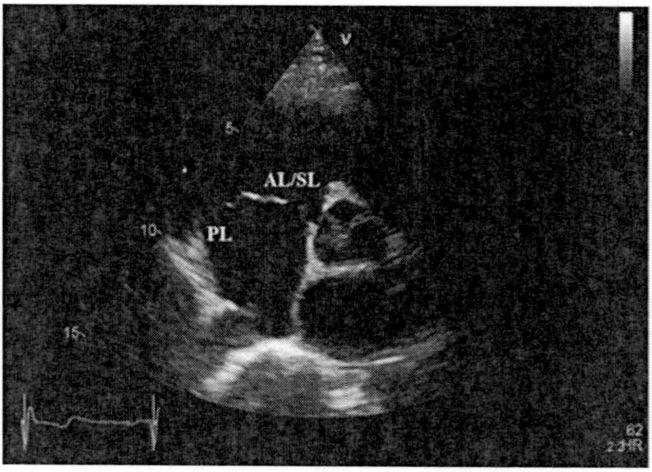

Figure 1B. Two-dimensional transthoracic echocardiography: parasternal short axis view. Rotating the probe of about 90 degrees from a parasternal long axis view, we find the tricuspid valve next to aortic right coronary cusp. AL = anterior leaflet; PL = posterior leaflet; SL = septal leaflet.

The flexibility of TTE is the possibility to visualize the structures through different projections.

In parasternal long axis view angling the probe down, thus directing the ultrasound beam toward the patient's right hip, the parasternal RV inflow long axis view is obtained (Figure 1A). The leaflet on the upper right side of the screen is the anterior one, on the bottom of the image there is the septal or the posterior leaflet according to the rotation of the probe (more or less vertically, about 15-25 degrees). Congenital or acquired abnormalities of TV leaflets are easily visible in this view that however it is not obtainable in every patient. It is not recommended to measure TA in this view for inaccurate geometrical assumptions.

In parasternal short axis view at aortic level, TV is placed transversely to right coronary aortic cusp (Figure 1B), being nearly vertical, at approximately 45° to sagittal plane. The septal leaflet can be seen near the right coronary artery ostium or trajectory; angling the probe more anteriorly, at the same level, the anterior leaflet is visualized. On the opposite side, the posterior leaflet is reached. Subvalvular apparatus and the inlet portion of the right ventricle can be clearly and accurately seen with this projection.

In the apical four-chambers view, (Figure 2), septal and anterior leaflets can be evaluated focusing the ultrasound beam on the right heart (tilting the probe towards the sternum). Moreover, this is the best view to measure TA and the recommended one to confirm the indication for TV repair [5], due a lower interobserver variability in comparison to other views [4]. Annulus fractional shortening is here calculated using the distance between the insertion of anterior and septal leaflets at end-diastole and at end-systole. The longitudinal systolic excursion of the tricuspid annulus (TAPSE), measured in mono-dimensional mode placing the cursor at the insertion of the anterior leaflet on RV free wall, is a paramount index of RV function, with diagnostic and prognostic purposes.

The apical two chamber view is obtained rotating the probe about 90 degrees from the apical four-chambers view; the image outlines the right ventricle along the major axis and allow the evaluation of the posterior and anterior leaflet.

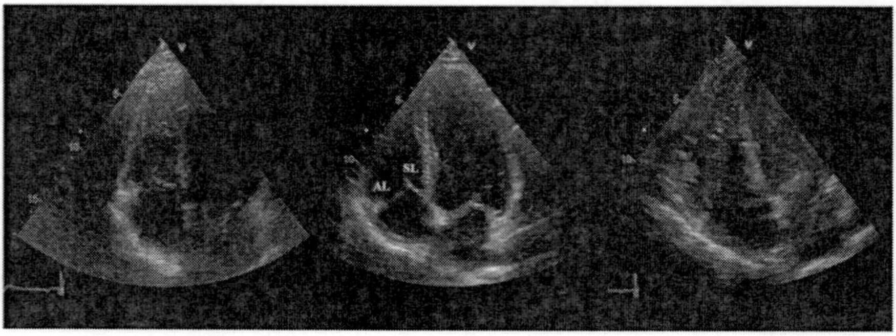

Figure 2. Two-dimensional transthoracic echocardiography: apical four chambers view. Moving the probe from a conventional four chambers view (central image) to a medial (left image) or lateral (right image) position, anterior (AL) and septal (SL) leaflets can be evaluated. This is also the recommended view to measure the tricuspid annulus.

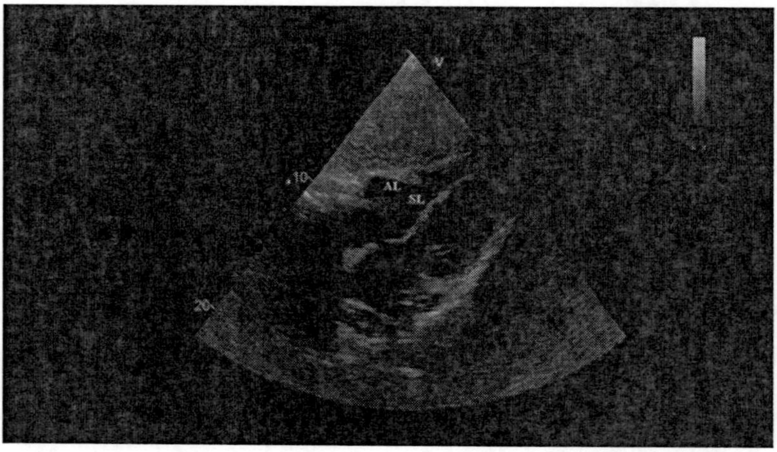

Figure 3. Two-dimensional transthoracic echocardiography: subcostal four chambers view. AL = anterior leaflet; SL = septal leaflet.

The subcostal view is an extremely useful way to assess TV in patients with poor parasternal and apical acoustic windows. The *standard subcostal four-chambers view* allows to visualize the anterior and septal leaflet (Figure 3), while in *short axis* the posterior leaflet is better visualized along with the anterior or the septal leaflet. Interestingly, rotating the probe 90 degrees from the subcostal four-chambers view, it is possible to appreciate the three leaflets at the same time, the so called "en face" view: the anterior leaflet is shown on the upper left side of the screen, the posterior leaflet on the upper right side and the septal leaflet at the bottom of the acquired image.

Doppler Evaluation of the Tricuspid Valve

As mentioned at the beginning of the chapter, a complete evaluation of the tricuspid valve cannot be performed without continuous wave (CW) or color flow mapping (CFM) analysis. An abnormality of the annulus, of one or more leaflets, chordae tendineae or papillary muscles, but also of the right atrium and ventricle may result in valve malfunction.

The tricuspid valve stenosis is a rare entity at our latitudes; the main etiologies include: rheumatic heart disease, congenital stenosis, right atrial tumors, carcinoid heart disease and endocarditis. The valve apparatus usually shows thickening or calcifications with restricted diastolic mobility and right atrial dilatation.

The detection of high velocities during diastole with color aliasing, usually associated with a certain degree of regurgitation, are typical of tricuspid stenosis. For better evaluation, a four-chamber apical projection focused on the right heart or a long axis parasternal projection in which the right inflow is visualized is recommended [6].

Tricuspid flow is conditioned by respiratory movements, so each measure is best evaluated at end-expiration or should be repeated during all the respiratory cycle and then averaged. Normal TV inflow velocity is up to 0.7 m/sec; usually TS is considered as a recorded velocity of >1 m/s during expiration but can reach >2 m/s during inspiration [7]. Significant TS, with or without associated TR is characterized by a mean pressure gradient of >5 mmHg and an inflow time-velocity integral of >60 cm [6]. A cut-off value for Pressure Half Time (PHT) of ≥190 ms has been proposed, but is poorly accurate [7]. Also, the finding of a high right atrial volume and a dilated and non-collapsible inferior vena cava support the diagnosis of tricuspid stenosis.

When assessing the tricuspid valve regurgitation it is necessary to remember a physiopathological distinction that has morpho-functional bases, i.e., the primary and secondary insufficiency [8]. Primary TR is due to an intrinsic defect of the valve; functional TR is secondary to other heart pathologies including left heart ventricular dysfunction or valve diseases, pulmonary hypertension and RV dysfunction, as in myocardial infarction or pulmonary embolism [9].

A trivial or mild TR can be considered as a normal finding in general population, with a prevalence of 15% of men and 18% of women in the Framingham study [10]. Being mostly asymptomatic, TR is often an occasional evidence. Functional TR is the most prevalent type, about 75% of all TR, and is characterized by annular dilatation, mostly in septo-lateral direction, and leaflets tethering [11]. The apical displacement of the leaflets can be quantified in apical 4 chambers view by measuring tenting area (that is the area between TV annulus and TV leaflets in mid-systole) and coaptation depth (the distance between TV annulus plane and the point of coaptation of the leaflets at the same point of the cardiac cycle). A tenting area over 1 cm^2 indicates severe TR [12].

A correct assessment of valve regurgitation requires qualitative and quantitative methods. Color Doppler is the first and easiest tool to identify the presence of TR and allows the application of key parameters to quantify regurgitation severity: identifies the origin of the regurgitant jet and its direction, assess the flow convergence, estimates the vena contracta (VC) width and the jet area. All these indexes should be assessed in apical four chambers view [13]. The flow converge proximally to the TR orifice is useful both to identify the location of the valve abnormality and to understand the magnitude of regurgitation [14]. In fact, the largest and the more persistent is the flow convergence, the more severe is the valve regurgitation. Regurgitant jet area is highly dependent on color velocity scale and gain but also on the hemodynamic state of the patient. Moreover, in case of very severe TR, it underestimates the real grade of the regurgitation. The VC width is a semiquantitative method, defined as the narrowest portion of the regurgitant flow that occurs at or immediately downstream of the regurgitant orifice [15]. It is less pressure-dependent even if, in functional TR, the patient's volume load might influence the orifice size. A reduction of color sector and a zoomed view are essential for a more precise measurement which is also subordinate to a correct ultrasound beam orientation, often difficult in TR. Quantitative methods include effective regurgitant orifice area (EROA) and regurgitant fraction that can be quite easily obtained by proximal isovelocity surface area (PISA) method. PISA is based on the concept that the blood flow, while approaching the regurgitant orifice, increases its velocity in concentric shells recognizable by color Doppler. The first key step is to reduce color aliasing velocity (Av) up to 20-40 cm/sec. We can then measure the radius of the hemisphere of the flow convergence at peak TR velocity. The latter is also a component of EROA calculation according to the formula:

$$2\pi r^2 \times Av \times PeakVofRjet$$

where r^2 is the PISA radius, Av the aliasing velocity of the color Doppler and PeakVofRjet the peak velocity of regurgitant jet obtained by CW Doppler. The EROA requires an optimal ultrasound beam alignment and is more complicated than qualitative methods but it is considered as the best parameter for the quantification of TR. Multiplying EROA for the velocity-time integral (VTI) of the tricuspid regurgitation by CW Doppler we get the regurgitant volume. CW Doppler is useful not only for EROA and regurgitant volume measurement but also to acquire more information on TR severity. Usually the spectral density of the regurgitant flow helps in the identification of mild insufficiency when incomplete and faint, while being less reliable in moderate-to-severe jets. Nevertheless, it is dependent on jet direction (central vs eccentric) for the different alignment. The duration of the parabolic curve of the jet is an index of hemodynamic impact during RV systole. As for mitral valve, in case of a functional TR limited to the phases of isovolumic contraction and relaxation, the magnitude of the regurgitation is mild [16]. CW Doppler is also helpful for the estimation of pulmonary artery systolic pressure. The presence of reverse flow at hepatic veins by Pulsed Wave (PW) Doppler is a specific but scarcely sensitive index of severe TR.

Severe TR is defined by the European Society of CardioVascular Imaging (EACVI) [13], in presence of abnormalities of the TV and one or more between:

- Very large central or eccentric, especially if the jet has high density and a triangular shape with early peaking;
- VC >7 mm;
- PISA radius > 9 mm;
- EROA ≥40 mm^2;
- Regurgitant volume ≥45 ml

The consensus of the EACVI suggests advocating severity of TR by using VC width and PISA radius in apical four chambers view, except in the presence of trivial or mild TR.

According to 2017 ESC guidelines [5], the treatment approach to TR is different whether the patient also requires left heart surgery or not. In the first case, if secondary TR is mild or moderate, TV repair is indicated only when TA is dilatated or signs of RV failure are evident; if TR is severe, repair is always indicated. When no left side operation is needed, a severe primary or secondary (in absence of left or RV dysfunction and severe pulmonary hypertension) TR should be repaired if the patients is strongly symptomatic or signs of RV dysfunction are developing. In conclusion, surgery is indicated, in class I with level of evidence C, in patients with severe primary TR undergoing left-sided valve surgery or with severe isolated primary TR without severe RV dysfunction, but also in patients with severe secondary TR undergoing left-sided valve surgery.

Up to 50% of patients operated for a mitral valve disease develops recurrent or persistent TR [17] and this seems to be related to pre-surgical RV dysfunction and severity of the TR. A dilated TA appears as one of the best predictors for this purpose [18]. On the contrary, a tenting area >1.63 cm^2 portends significant residual TR after TV annuloplasty [19].

Trans-Esophageal Echocardiography of the Tricuspid Valve

Although the TV is anatomically the most complex valve of the four cardiac valves, the incremental value of transesophageal echocardiography (TEE) for TV evaluation is lower than for the mitral valve [20]. This may be explained by the anterior position and thus greater distance from the probe of the TV as compared to the mitral valve, usually making TTE the method of choice in the clinical and preoperative scenario. However, technically adequate and complete TTE examination may be difficult in some patients. These include the obese, those with hyper-inflated lungs (such as patients with chronic obstructive pulmonary disease), intubated patients, and those who cannot be optimally positioned, such as patients post cardiac surgery. Furthermore, TEE evaluation is of utmost interest for the diagnosis of endocarditis, venous catheters and pacemaker lead infections, and visualization of traumatic rupture of the TV and it is fundamental for intraoperative monitoring [21] during percutaneous intervention [22].

Transesophageal Echocardiographic Views for the Tricuspid Valve

The evaluation of the tricuspid valve by the TEE technique is structured through four distinct projections: mid-esophageal four-chamber view; mid-esophageal RV inflow-outflow view; mid-esophageal modified bicaval view; transgastric views [23–25]. Below is a schematic description of the acquisition method and the technical part relating to the individual projections:

Mid-esophageal four-chamber view: to optimize the TV view a slight clockwise (rightward) rotation from the typical four-chamber view (Figure 4A) usually allows to move the TV to the center of the scan, and to visualize the septal leaflet on the right and the anterior or posterior leaflet on the left, depending on the amount of anteflexion or retroflexion of the probe (Figure 4B). Advancing or withdrawing the transducer allows to image the entire TV.

Mid-esophageal RV inflow-outflow view: starting from the mid-esophageal four chamber view and rotating the angle forward to around 30-60° will produce a cross-sectional view of the aortic valve with a transverse section of the RV inflow and outflow tracts (Figure 4C). This view allows to set the probe to obtain a nearly orthogonal view of the TV and thus to optimize the assessment of quantitative measurements of TV flow velocities. In this view, the anterior or the septal leaflet (depending on probe rotation) are next to the aortic valve, the posterior leaflet is on the left of the display.

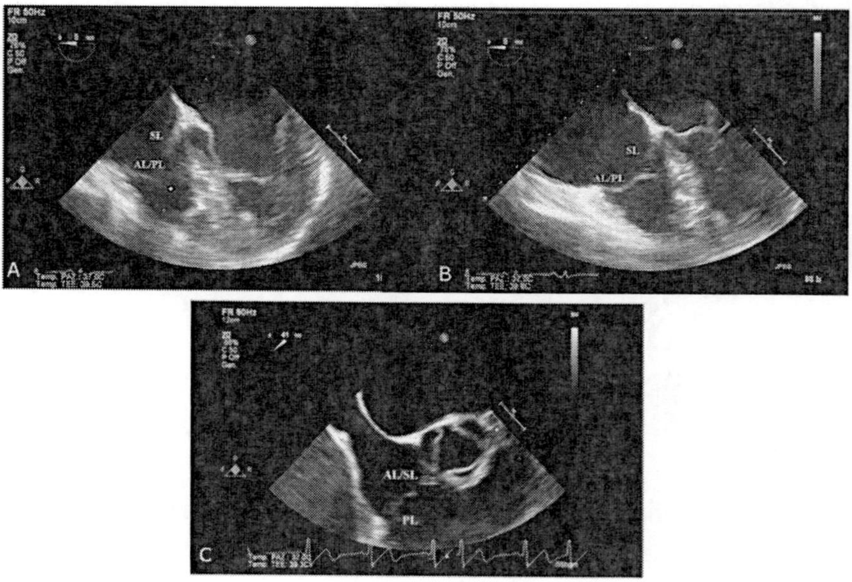

Figure 4. A: Two-dimensional transesophageal echocardiography: mid esophageal four-chambers view. It is obtained at 0° degrees. Tricuspid value is seen on the left. B: Two-dimensional transesophageal echocardiography: mid esophageal four-chambers view focused on right heart. A slight clockwise rotation of the probe from the conventional four-chambers view allows to optimize the evaluation of the tricuspid valve. C: Two-dimensional transesophageal echocardiography: mid esophageal right ventricular inflow-outflow view. At 30-60°, the tricuspid valve is seen in the lower left side of the aortic valve. AL = anterior leaflet; PL = posterior leaflet; SL = septal leaflet.

Mid-esophageal modified bicaval view: from the standard bicaval view (120 degrees) the omniplane angle should be increased until the TV appears in the far left of the display. This view usually provides the best alignment of the ultrasound beam and the TV regurgitation jet for continuous or pulsed Doppler measurements, especially in the case of eccentric regurgitant jets toward the interatrial septum, which often occurs since the septal leaflet has the shortest radial length and is most often fixed by the rigid TA.

Transgastric views: from the transgastric view of the left ventricle a clockwise (rightward) rotation allows to obtain a good view of the TV in short axis (30°), identifying the septal (right sided), anterior (left sided, far field) and posterior leaflets (left sided, near field). A long axis of the right ventricle is then obtained by rotating the multiplane angle to about 120°. The RV inflow view usually provides the best images for RV papillary muscles and chordae tendineae. The posterior leaflet of the TV is then visualized in the near field, attached to the inferior wall of the right ventricle, while the anterior leaflet is located in the far field, attached to the anterior wall of the right ventricle.

Whenever significant TV disease is seen on echocardiogram, concomitant assessment of the right heart must ensue. As for the right ventricle, *three views are similar to those used for TV evaluation*: the mid-esophageal four chamber view, the mid-esophageal inflow-outflow view and the transgastric views, the latter obtained at mid-papillary and RV inflow levels in short-axis or with the whole right ventricle in long-axis view. Likewise, the right atrium may be scanned at the mid esophageal four chamber and inflow-outflow views, as well as through the mid esophageal bicaval view.

Transesophageal Doppler Evaluation of the Tricuspid Valve

As already explained, Color Doppler imaging is key to quantify the severity of tricuspid stenosis (TS) and tricuspid regurgitation (TR).

Assessment of the Tricuspid Stenosis

Rheumatic disease leads to thickening of the leaflets and commissural fusion as well as involvement of the subvalvular apparatus, which is usually better visualized at TEE especially in the transgastric long-axis view [24]. Other causes of TS include endomyocardial fibrosis, potentially associated with RV dysfunction and thrombosis, and carcinoid heart disease, with leaflets fixed in semi-open position and invariably associated with TV regurgitation [24].

Doppler evaluation is fundamental to establish TS severity [7, 24, 26]. The mid-esophageal RV inflow-outflow view is commonly used for CW Doppler estimation of TS: assessment of the diastolic pressure gradients using CW Doppler can be performed while increasing the sweep speed (100 mm/s) to increase the accuracy of measurements. The PHT can be used to estimate the orifice area but is less well validated as compared to mitral stenosis. Conversely, in the absence of regurgitation, dividing the stroke volume measured at either the left or RV outflow tract by the tricuspid inflow VTI from the CW Doppler recording (continuity equation) can be used to calculate the stenotic orifice area.

In addition, planimetry of the valvular orifice in the transgastric short-axis view can be attempted, but it is difficult and unlikely to yield accurate results [24].

Assessment of the Tricuspid Regurgitation

TEE examination of the tricuspid valve apparatus may provide significant information regarding the underlying cause and mechanism of tricuspid regurgitation. The three leaflets of the TV are not simultaneously visualized in 2D assessment and thus a combination of different views usually allows the evaluation of the subvalvular apparatus, right atrium and right ventricle. Most commonly, TR is due to RV dilation/dysfunction due to pulmonary hypertension or RV infarction. Although the measurement of the TA should be done in multiple views (during diastole), the measurement from the transgastric RV inflow long-axis view correlates best with surgical measurements [27]. Rheumatic heart disease and carcinoid heart disease result in thickening, restricted mobility of the leaflets, while endocarditis may cause destruction of the leaflets and/or chordae. In the Ebstein's anomaly a displacement index may be calculated in the midesophageal four-chamber view, as the distance between the two hinge points of the septal leaflet relative to that of the anterior mitral leaflet indexed to body surface area (>8 mm/m^2) [24, 28].

In TEE, the multiplane angle should be optimized to obtain the largest possible jet of regurgitation. The VC is usually measured in the mid-esophageal four chamber view, which is also helpful for jet area estimation in the case of centrally directed regurgitation, whereas it is less informative in the case of eccentric jets or multiple jets [13, 24, 28]. In the same view, it is also possible to quantitatively calculate the EROA and the regurgitant volume, through the PISA method, as already explained above [13], once the basic assumption for its application (circularity of regurgitant orifice) are met, which often does not apply for secondary TR. On the other hand, the inflow velocity and the quality of CW Doppler (dense, triangular, early peaking) of TR are best imaged in the mid esophageal RV inflow-outflow view or alternatively in the modified bicaval view [30].

Using CW Doppler, measurement of the peak tricuspid regurgitation jet velocity can be performed to estimate pulmonary artery pressure [13]. Usually, the midesophageal RV inflow-outflow view provides good alignment of the regurgitation jet with the Doppler signal [24]. Localization of the jet is assisted by color Doppler flow mapping, and angulation of the probe with adjustment of the multiplane angle should be performed in order to identify the maximal velocity jet. To obtain the right atrial pressure, as in TTE, the respirophasic changes in the diameter of the inferior vena cava (IVC) should be evaluated, usually in the bicaval view. In case of mechanically ventilated patients, the ventilator should be turned off at the time of the measurement and a specific equation proposed by Arthur and colleagues may be applied:

right atrial pressure = [inferior vena cava diameter - 4.004/0.751 [29]

Imaging of the hepatic veins can be obtained by the transgastric position withdrawing the probe and rotating it to the right to visualize liver parenchyma in the transverse plane. The hepatic veins can be identified with the help of color Doppler, with PW Doppler used to assess the presence of reverse systolic flow, as index of TR severity. Likewise, from the mid esophageal four chamber view by advancing and slightly retroflexing the probe it is possible to image the long-axis of the coronary sinus. Again, a reversal systolic flow in the coronary sinus is an index of TR severity [30].

Transesophageal Echocardiography in Endocarditis, Venous Catheters and Pacemaker Lead Infections

Right-sided endocarditis is common in intravenous drug users, in patients with implantable cardiac devices, right heart congenital abnormalities or concomitant left-sided endocarditis [31]. The European guidelines consider TEE as the first-line imaging modality in suspected infective endocarditis, even in cases of positive results at TTE [32]. Its superiority in the diagnosis of periannular complications and measurement of vegetation size, both important parameters to plan the therapeutic strategy, has been extensively demonstrated. Moreover, TEE offers crucial prognostic information, although most of these evidences mainly apply to left-sided endocarditis [31, 32]. Right-sided endocarditis usually involve the TV, are larger, have fewer periannular complications, lead more often to pulmonary thromboembolism and have better outcomes as compared to left-sided endocarditis.

The TEE examination must include the *mid-esophageal four-chamber view* and *RV inflow-outflow view* (to also assess the pulmonary valve), the *gastric short-axis and long-axis view* (for subvalvular apparatus), the *bicaval view and the frontal long-axis view of the coronary sinus* [31].

It was demonstrated that TTE and TEE have similar diagnostic accuracy in drug abusers [33], since patients are usually younger and with good TTE windows and right-sided vegetation are larger and closer to the TTE probe than the TEE one. However, in some cases TEE still performs better than TTE, such as poor acoustic TTE windows, suspected concomitant pulmonary valve or left sided endocarditis, presence of central catheters, in case of negative results on TTE and moderate/high clinical suspicion or when an alternative diagnosis is lacking. Right-sided endocarditis can affect patients with right-heart congenital abnormalities. This condition is rare in adults and has been comprehensive reviewed in [34].

However, the main advantage of TEE over TTE mainly lies in patients with implanted cardiac devices. Indeed, vegetations are frequently located at the level of the upper part of the right atrium and even into the superior vena cava (SVC), and both are areas better targeted with TEE than TTE (38). Furthermore, patients with cardiac devices are older and have inadequate acoustic windows and intracardiac leads induce reverberations and artifacts that hinder the identification of a vegetation. A few studies have compared the diagnostic accuracy of TTE and TEE in this setting, finding an overall sensitivity of 25 and 84%, respectively [35, 36].

Finally, the role of TTE and TEE in patients who are not intravenous drug users, without implanted cardiac devices, or congenital heart disease, the "three no's" endocarditis group, has not been assessed, but usually this group shares epidemiologic and clinical characteristics with intravenous drug abusers. On the other hand, many of these patients have central lines (lower performance of TTE) and/or higher comorbidities/more aggressive microbiologic profiles, thus often deserving a TEE approach.

3D Transesophageal Echocardiography

The TV plane is usually not coaxial with TEE imaging plane, making difficult a simultaneous assessment of all the three TV leaflets with two-dimensional TEE.

Conversely, three-dimensional TEE allows to scan all components of the TV using a single full-volume data set or to perform a focused examination on a particular TV detail using a narrower imaging acquisition mode with higher resolution [1, 24, 25].

Acquisition is usually done from a 0° to a 30° view in the midesophageal four chamber view, with the TV centered in the image, or alternatively with a 40° transgastric view with anteflexion. The septal leaflet should be located in the 6 o'clock position when displaying the TV en face [25]. These views may be of incremental diagnostic value in case of leaflet prolapse, perforation, or vegetation, as well as to identify regurgitation jets, or to trace planimetry of the tricuspid orifice area to assess the TS severity. To visualize a particular section of the TV the cropping plane can be adjusted.

Wide-angle acquisition mode allows visualization of the whole TV apparatus. from the annulus to the papillary muscle tips. The loss of temporal resolution associate with wide-angle acquisition can be ameliorated using multiple-beat mode, which also increases spatial resolution [1, 25].

Color flow Doppler should be also acquired in patients with TR and/or TS, after the identification of a region of interest in the orthogonal planes, which should be limited to the TV apparatus and color flow Doppler jet to optimize the frame rate. A lower line density will permit a larger sector to be displayed.

The 3D TTE and 3D TEE seems to provide a comparable visualization of the shape and dimension of the TV annulus and a simultaneous visualization of the three leaflets [37]. However, 3D TEE seems to be less dependent than 3D TTE on the acoustic window and less impaired by blurring artifacts leading to leaflet thickness overestimation [38]. Moreover, 3D TTE seems to yield the best view of leaflet papillary muscles and chordae from the transgastric view [37].

Transesophageal Echocardiography in Tricuspid Valve Surgery

In the last decade, TEE has become the mainstay in valve repair surgery. Whit regards to TV, TEE allows intraoperative quantification of TR and helps defying the intraoperative surgical strategy as well as the evaluation of surgical results.

Most of the TEE driven intraoperative decisions on TV are made in the context of mitral valve disease, either regurgitation or stenosis. In facts, it was demonstrated that the prognosis of patients in which TV regurgitation was left untreated was considerably worse than those in which the valve was repaired [21].

First of all, intraoperative TEE is useful to calibrate the right surgical plan upon each single patient. In fact, Bajzer et al. demonstrated that in patients undergoing intraoperative TEE the surgical plan was modified in about 10% of the cases based upon echocardiographic findings [39]. In addition to that, intraoperative TEE ensured a more accurate estimation of residual 3+ or 4+ TR, allowing for further correction in the same thoracotomy. However, no effect was demonstrated about the use of intraoperative TEE on long-term mortality.

Among the parameters evaluated with intraoperative TEE, TA diameter is usually considered the most reliable predictor of TR persistence after surgical interventions. In fact, the TR jet is based on a velocity map rather than a volume map, and it is therefore dependent upon loading conditions. Therefore, under general anesthesia, the effective regurgitant jet might be underestimated, leading to potential under treatment of the TV [21].

Tricuspid valve diameter, on the other hand, has been consistently shown to predict reversibility of TR after cardiac surgery [21]. In fact, when annuloplasty was performed regardless of TR in presence of a septolateral diameter of the TA > 40 mm, survival rates where greater than those in which annuloplasty was not performed (90.3% vs 85.5% survival rate at 10 years). Nowadays, there is large consensus that TV annuloplasty should be performed regardless of TR in presence of a TA > 40 mm, or > 21 mm/m2 of body surface or in case of an intraoperative annulus > 70 mm (corresponding to an echocardiographic annulus of 40 mm) [40]. There is less consensus about the TA target dimensions in TV repair; some authors have suggested a correction up to normal values of 30 mm, and the most common ring size used are between 28 and 30 mm for the Cosgrove-Edwards rings and between 30 mm and 32 mm for the Carpentier-Edwards rings [41].

The Cleveland Clinic group has shown that increased preoperative tricuspid leaflet tethering height and area, low left ventricular ejection fraction and increased RV pressure were related to worse TR during follow up, and predicted early and mid-term adverse outcomes of ring annuloplasty [42]. Thus, patients with significant tethering, significant distortion of the valve, LV and RV dysfunction or severe pulmonary hypertension may require TV replacement to avoid long-term repair failure and adverse clinical outcomes.

The 3D TEE may provide incremental information and help to predict the outcome of TV surgery in functional TR. In fact, the TA is not only dilated, but also loses its axial dynamism and its non-planar shape, assuming a flatter disposition. Furthermore, in functional TR, the RV basal, mid and longitudinal diameters are significantly dilated. However, further studies are needed to confirm if those parameters have a prognostic significance in the setting of TV surgery beyond standard 2D TEE assessment [43].

Intraoperative TEE transesophageal echocardiogram can also be an "interventional" tool as it allows for further adjustment of the tension on the TA during annuloplasty.

In particular, TEE allows the achievement of minimal or no regurgitation in case of tricuspidal annuloplasty in 95% of the cases, as opposed to the 44% with manual palpation, avoiding reinstitution of cardiopulmonary bypass. No significant increase of peak inflow velocity and peak gradient was observed after TEE adjustment of tension, leading to no additional stenosis of the valve [44, 45].

Finally, intraoperative TEE may drive to a change in the original surgical plan also in cases of other valve surgeries or coronary artery bypass grafting. In fact, TEE allowed to omit or add TV repair in 0.16%, 0.2% and 1.8% of patients undergoing coronary artery bypass grafting, aortic valve replacement and mitral valve replacement/repair, respectively, in a retrospective analysis on 12.566 patients [46].

Transesophageal Echocardiography during the Tricuspid Valve Percutaneous Interventions

Nowadays, several percutaneous options for TV repair are available with bioprosthetic valves with: the MitraClip system (Abbott Vascular, Abbott Park, Illinois, USA); annular reduction techniques (Tricinch device, 4Tech Cardio, Galway, Ireland); transcatheter bicuspidalization (Trialign device, Mitralign, Boston, Massachusetts, USA); direct annuloplasty using the Cardioband device (Valtech Cardio, Or Yehuda, Israel); leaflet coaptation systems using the Transcatheter Forma Repair System (Edwards Lifesciences, Irvine, California, USA) [46, 47].

The percutaneous implantation of a bioprosthesis in the tricuspid position is one of the most challenging. In fact, the anatomy and dimensions of the TA, the lower pressures of the RV chamber, its trabeculae and the anatomy of the TA in relation to the IVC and SVC make the procedure extremely difficult, so that its feasibility has been demonstrated for valve in valve procedures (in case of degenerated surgical bioprosthesis) and valve in ring procedures (in case of failed annuloplasty) [48].

With the advent of percutaneous procedures, multimodality imaging has become crucial to carry out the intervention. Even though TTE could be, at least sometimes, sufficient for the imaging of the TV during percutaneous interventions, the multiple planes of view obtained with TEE offer a great advantage to the operator. Intraoperative TEE, in fact, is an imaging technique that does not require interruption for catheters and wires repositioning, and that allows their visualization throughout the procedure [48].

The first devices tested were the bioprosthesis placed in the IVC and SVC under echocardiographic guidance, which allowed the visualization of the junction between the right atrium and the SVC in the mid-esophageal view, and the imaging of the IVC and the hepatic veins in the transgastirc views [22, 47, 48].

For what concerns the MitraClip device, low esophageal views allow the detection of the clip and its positioning as perpendicular as possible to the beam for optimal positioning. Moreover, low esophageal views also allow the detection of residual regurgitation and leaflet grasp, and allow the detection of the transvalvular gradient (with a maximum acceptable gradient of 3 mmHg). Deep transgastric views are also useful to assess the correct positioning of the clips.

Moving to the Forma Spacer device, a leaflet coaptation anchor system, transgastric views are essential for the detection of the optimal RV sites for anchoring, while mid-esophageal views are essential for the assessment of the vena contracta and the measurement of the dimensions of the implantable prosthesis. Moreover, in those views the effective TR can be measured and, by means of 3D TEE, the results can be assessed after device placement [22, 48].

With the Trialign system, that allows the bicuspidalization of the TV similar to a modified Kay procedure, intraoperative TEE imaging is essential. In fact, mid and deep esophageal windows allow for the correct positioning of the wires beneath the tricuspidal annulus, between the posterior and septal leaflet commissures, avoiding the right coronary artery and the base of the leaflet itself. After correct wires placement, continuous TEE imaging allows for the detection of the positions of the pledgets sutures until maximum annular reduction is achieved. Finally, postoperative 3D imaging allows for the reconstruction of the newly formed annulus and for the measurement of the EROA [48].

Conclusion

The complexity of the tricuspid valve requires a multimodal approach for its evaluation. TTE and TEE echocardiography, associated with 3D techniques, allow accurate anatomical visualization; not secondarily, these acquisitions take place in full hemodynamic load, increasing the value of the acquired data. These methods, for their diffusion and flexibility of use (outpatient, pre- and intra-operative assessment and follow-up evaluation) constitute the core of the image of the tricuspid valve in current practice. On them the clinician guides the medical therapy and surgical timing, the surgeon plans the most appropriate intervention and displays the result, whether it is performed with traditional surgery or with new trans-catheter approaches.

References

[1] Lang RM, Badano LP, Tsang (2012). EAE/ASE Recommendations for Image Acquisition and Display Using Three-Dimensional Echocardiography. *Eur Heart J - Cardiovasc Imaging* 13:1–46.

[2] Ton-Nu T-T, Levine RA, Handschumacher MD, Dorer DJ, Yosefy C, Fan D, Hua L, Jiang L, Hung J (2006). Geometric Determinants of Functional Tricuspid Regurgitation. *Circulation* 114:143–149.

[3] Fukuda S (2006). Three-Dimensional Geometry of the Tricuspid Annulus in Healthy Subjects and in Patients With Functional Tricuspid Regurgitation: A Real-Time, 3-Dimensional Echocardiographic Study. *Circulation* 114:I–492–I–498.

[4] Anwar AM, Geleijnse ML, Cate FJ, Meijboom FJ (2006). Assessment of tricuspid valve annulus size, shape and function using real-time three-dimensional echocardiography. *Interact Cardiovasc Thorac Surg* 5:683–687.

[5] Baumgartner H, Falk V, Bax J (2017). 2017 ESC/EACTS guidelines for the management of valvular heart disease. *Eur Heart J* 38:2739–2791.

[6] Baumgartner H, Hung J, Bermejo J, Chambers JB, Evangelista A, Griffin BP, Iung B, Otto CM, Pellikka PA, Quinones M (2009). Echocardiographic assessment of valve stenosis: EAE/ASE recommendations for clinical practice. *Eur J Echocardiogr* 10:1–25.

[7] Fawzy ME, Mercer EN, Dunn B, al-Amri M, Andaya W (1989). Doppler echocardiography in the evaluation of tricuspid stenosis. *Eur Heart J* 10:985–990.

[8] Huttin O, Voilliot D, Mandry D, Venner C, Juillière Y, Selton-Suty C (2016). All you need to know about the tricuspid valve: tricuspid

valve imaging and tricuspid regurgitation analysis. *Arch Cardiovasc Dis* 109:67–80.

[9] Rogers JH, Bolling SF (2009). The tricuspid valve: Current perspective and evolving management of tricuspid regurgitation. *Circulation* 119:2718–2725.

[10] Singh JP, Evans JC, Levy D, Larson MG, Freed LA, Fuller DL, Lehman B, Benjamin EJ (1999). Prevalence and clinical determinants of mitral, tricuspid, and aortic regurgitation (The Framingham Heart Study). *Am J Cardiol* 83:897–902.

[11] Spinner EM, Shannon P, Buice D, Jimenez JH, Veledar E, Nido PJ del, Adams DH, Yoganathan AP (2011). In Vitro Characterization of the Mechanisms Responsible for Functional Tricuspid Regurgitation. *Circulation* 124:920–929.

[12] Kim H-K, Kim Y-J, Park J-S, Kim KH, Kim K-B, Ahn H, Sohn D-W, Oh B-H, Park Y-B, Choi Y-S (2006). Determinants of the Severity of Functional Tricuspid Regurgitation. *Am J Cardiol* 98:236–242.

[13] Lancellotti P, Tribouilloy C, Hagendorff A, Popescu BA, Edvardsen T, Pierard LA, Badano L, and JLZ (2013). Recommendations for the echocardiographic assessment of native valvular regurgitation: an executive summary from the European Association of Cardiovascular Imaging. *Eur Heart J - Cardiovasc Imaging* 14:611–644.

[14] Bargiggia GS, Tronconi L, Sahn DJ, Recusani F, Raisaro A, Servi SD, Valdes-Cruz LM, Montemartini C (1991). A new method for quantitation of mitral regurgitation based on color flow Doppler imaging of flow convergence proximal to regurgitant orifice. *Circulation* 84:1481–1489.

[15] Zoghbi WA, Adams D, Bonow RO, et al. (2017). Recommendations for Noninvasive Evaluation of Native Valvular Regurgitation. *J Am Soc Echocardiogr* 30:303–371.

[16] Schwammenthal E, Chen C, Benning F, Block M, Breithardt G, Levine RA (1994). Dynamics of mitral regurgitant flow and orifice area. Physiologic application of the proximal flow convergence

method: clinical data and experimental testing. *Circulation* 90:307–322.

[17] Matsunaga A, Duran CMG (2005). Progression of tricuspid regurgitation after repaired functional ischemic mitral regurgitation. *Circulation* 112:I453-457.

[18] Badano LP, Muraru D, Enriquez-Sarano M (2013). Assessment of functional tricuspid regurgitation. *Eur Heart J* 34:1875–1885.

[19] Fukuda S (2006). Determinants of Recurrent or Residual Functional Tricuspid Regurgitation after Tricuspid Annuloplasty. *Circulation* 114:I–582–I–587.

[20] Luxford J, Bassin L, D'Ambra M (2017). Echocardiography of the tricuspid valve. *Ann Cardiothorac Surg* 6:223–239.

[21] Montealegre-Gallegos M, Bergman R, Jiang L, Matyal R, Mahmood B, Mahmood F (2014). Tricuspid Valve: An Intraoperative Echocardiographic Perspective. *J Cardiothorac Vasc Anesth* 28:761–770.

[22] Ancona F, Stella S, Taramasso M (2017). Multimodality imaging of the tricuspid valve with implication for percutaneous repair approaches. *Heart* 103:1073–1081.

[23] Perrino AC, Reeves ST (2013). *A practical Approach to Transesophageal Echocardiography*, 3rd ed. Lippincott Williams and Wilkins, Philadelphia – USA.

[24] Mathew JP, Swaminathan M, Ayoub CM (2010). *Clinical manual and review of transesophageal echochardiography.,* 2nd ed. McGraw-Hill, USA.

[25] Hahn RT, Abraham T, Adams MS (2013). Guidelines for Performing a Comprehensive Transesophageal Echocardiographic Examination: Recommendations from the American Society of Echocardiography and the Society of Cardiovascular Anesthesiologists. *J Am Soc Echocardiogr* 26:921–964.

[26] Karp K, Teien D, Eriksson P (1989). Doppler echocardiographic assessment of the valve area in patients with atrioventricular valve stenosis by application of the continuity equation. *J Intern Med* 225:261–266.

[27] Maslow AD, Schwartz C, Singh AK (2004). Assessment of the tricuspid valve: A comparison of four transesophageal echocardiographic windows. *J Cardiothorac Vasc Anesth* 18:719–724.

[28] Ammash NM, Warnes CA, Connolly HM, Danielson GK, Seward JB (1997). Mimics of Ebstein's anomaly. *Am Heart J* 134:508–513.

[29] Arthur ME, Landolfo C, Wade M, Castresana MR (2009). Inferior Vena Cava Diameter (IVCD) Measured with Transesophageal Echocardiography (TEE) Can Be Used to Derive the Central Venous Pressure (CVP) in Anesthetized Mechanically Ventilated Patients. *Echocardiography* 26:140–149.

[30] Zamorano J, Almeria C, Alfonso F, Perez MA, Grauper C, Morales R, Sanchez-Harguindey L (1997). Transesophageal Doppler Analysis of Coronary Sinus Flow A New Method to Assess the Severity of Tricuspid Regurgitation. *Echocardiography* 14:579–588.

[31] San Román JA, Vilacosta I, López J, Revilla A, Arnold R, Sevilla T, Rollán MJ (2012). Role of transthoracic and transesophageal echocardiography in right-sided endocarditis: one echocardiographic modality does not fit all. *J Am Soc Echocardiogr Off Publ Am Soc Echocardiogr* 25:807–814.

[32] Habib G (2009). Guidelines on the prevention, diagnosis, and treatment of infective endocarditis (new version 2009) The Task Force on the Prevention, Diagnosis, and Treatment of Infective Endocarditis of the European Society of Cardiology (ESC). *Eur Heart J* 30:2369–2413.

[33] Román JS, Vilacosta I, Zamorano J, Almería C, Sánchez-Harguindey L (1993). Transesophageal echocardiography in right-sided endocarditis. *J Am Coll Cardiol* 21:1226–1230.

[34] Di Filippo S (2006). Current patterns of infective endocarditis in congenital heart disease. *Heart* 92:1490–1495.

[35] Klug D, Lacroix D, Savoye C, Goullard L, Grandmougin D, Hennequin JL, Kacet S, Lekieffre J (1997). Systemic Infection Related to Endocarditis on Pacemaker Leads. *Circulation* 95:2098–2107.

[36] Victor F, Place CD, Camus C, Breton HL, Leclercq C, Pavin D, Mabo P, Daubert C (1999). Pacemaker lead infection: echocardiographic features, management, and outcome. *Heart* 81:82–87.

[37] Faletra FF, Leo LA, Paiocchi VL, Schlossbauer SA, Borruso MG, Pedrazzini G, Moccetti T, Ho SY (2018). Imaging-based tricuspid valve anatomy by computed tomography, magnetic resonance imaging, two and three-dimensional echocardiography: correlation with anatomic specimen. *Eur Heart J - Cardiovasc Imaging* 20:1–13.

[38] Faletra FF, Ramamurthi A, Dequarti MC, Leo LA, Moccetti T, Pandian N (2014). Artifacts in three-dimensional transesophageal echocardiography. *J Am Soc Echocardiogr Off Publ Am Soc Echocardiogr* 27:453–462.

[39] Bajzer CT, Stewart WJ, Cosgrove DM, Azzam SJ, Arheart KL, Klein AL (1998). Tricuspid valve surgery and intraoperative echocardiography: factors affecting survival, clinical outcome, and echocardiographic success. *J Am Coll Cardiol* 32:1023–1031.

[40] Bianchi G, Solinas M, Bevilacqua S, Glauber M (2009). Which patient undergoing mitral valve surgery should also have the tricuspid repair? *Interact Cardiovasc Thorac Surg* 9:1009–1020.

[41] McCarthy PM, Bhudia SK, Rajeswaran J, Hoercher KJ, Lytle BW, Cosgrove DM, Blackstone EH (2004). Tricuspid valve repair: durability and risk factors for failure. *J Thorac Cardiovasc Surg* 127:674–685.

[42] Topilsky Y (2015). Indications for Surgery for Tricuspid Regurgitation. *Interv Cardiol Rev* 10:58.

[43] Hai T, Amador Y, Mahmood F (2017). Changes in Tricuspid Annular Geometry in Patients with Functional Tricuspid Regurgitation. *J Cardiothorac Vasc Anesth* 31:2106–2114.

[44] De Simone R, Lange R, Tanzeem A, Gams E, Hagl S (1993). Adjustable tricuspid valve annuloplasty assisted by intraoperative transesophageal color Doppler echocardiography. *Am J Cardiol* 71:926–931.

[45] De Simone R, Lange R, Saggau W, Gams E, Tanzeem A, Hagl S (1992). Intraoperative transesophageal echocardiography for the evaluation of mitral, aortic and tricuspid valve repair \ast1A tool to optimize surgical outcome. *Eur J Cardiothorac Surg* 6:665–673.

[46] Eltzschig HK, Rosenberger P, Löffler M, Fox JA, Aranki SF, Shernan SK (2008). Impact of Intraoperative Transesophageal Echocardiography on Surgical Decisions in 12,566 Patients Undergoing Cardiac Surgery. *Ann Thorac Surg* 85:845–852.

[47] Hahn RT (2016). Transcathether Valve Replacement and Valve Repair. *Circ Res* 119:341–356.

[48] Hahn RT (2016). State-of-the-Art Review of Echocardiographic Imaging in the Evaluation and Treatment of Functional Tricuspid Regurgitation. *Circ Cardiovasc Imaging.* doi: 10.1161/circimaging. 116.005332.

In: The Rediscovered Tricuspid Valve ISBN: 978-1-53616-098-7
Editor: Giacomo Bianchi

Chapter 5

Advanced Imaging and Functional Tools for Tricuspid Valve Assessment: Cardiac MRI, CT-Scan and Cardiopulmonary Exercise Test

Giovanni Donato Aquaro[1,*], MD,
Alberto Clemente[1], MD,
Daniele Caratozzolo[2], MD
and Claudio Passino[1,2], MD, PhD
[1]Magnetic Resonance Imaging Unit,
Fondazione "G. Monasterio", Pisa, Italy
[2]Scuola Superiore Sant'Anna, Pisa, Italy

Abstract

Transthoracic and transesophageal echocardiograms are the most common non-invasive modalities for the diagnosis and quantification of tricuspid valve disease. Already today, thanks to the progress achieved in

* Corresponding Author's E-mail: aquaro@ftgm.it.

terms of speed of execution, access to resources, increased spatial and temporal resolution, third level imaging examinations such as MRI and CT scan are becoming the new protagonists of modern functional diagnostics. Their added value is to be able to combine the high-level image with the quantification of blood flows in order to further accurately define the valvular pathology. Even more recently, an already widely used instrument such as the Cardiopulmonary Exercise Test has increased its diagnostic accuracy through implementation with stress echocardiography, especially in right heart disease and in patients with out-of-proportion symptoms compared to resting hemodynamics.

Keywords: magnetic resonance, computed tomography, cardiopulmonary exercise test, tricuspid valve

INTRODUCTION

In the last two decades interest on tricuspid valve disease increased with the emerging evidences that functional tricuspid regurgitation is not an innocent bystander of mitral diseases, but rather an insidious condition leading to right heart failure and worse prognosis. Similarly, there is now an increasing awareness that correction of left-sided valvular disease would not result in a decrease of tricuspid regurgitation [1]. In patients with severe symptomatic tricuspid regurgitation medical therapy is often ineffective to improve symptoms and prognosis, while surgical therapy is effective to improve prognosis but is associated to high mortality and recurrence of regurgitation. Tricuspid annuloplasty in patients with moderate regurgitation and annular dilatation undergoing to left-sided surgery has demonstrated to be effective to prevent severe regurgitation without increasing the intraoperative mortality [2].

Echocardiography is the first line imaging technique to evaluate tricuspid anatomy and function; its information are often used as a sufficient tool for surgical planning and patient management.

However, in the next future third level imaging techniques as cardiac magnetic resonance (CMR) and computed tomography (CT) will guide clinical through the diagnostic and treatment planning phase of the disease, not only in case of suboptimal echocardiographic windows or to rule out disagreement between imaging modalities, but are also emerging as pivotal tool for transcatheter interventions [3].

A variety of cardiovascular diseases, including tricuspid valve diseases, are characterized by a reduced exercise tolerance: however, since fatigue, dyspnea and pain are all symptoms reported by patients, subjected to inter individual variability in reported intensity, an objective measure of exercise intolerance is required for a correct estimation of its severity. Cardiopulmonary exercise testing (CPET) is a test that has deeply changed the approach to assessment of exercise intolerance, linking physical performance to the underlying metabolic substratum and providing a highly reproducible evaluation of exercise capacity through various parameters. This functional test also allows to combine the results of the echocardiogram acquired at the same time to achieve a true CPET imaging in order to increase its diagnostic and prognostic value.

CARDIAC MAGNETIC RESONANCE

CMR is the gold standard imaging technique for the evaluation of cardiac function and soft tissue characterization. It provides high resolution dynamic images of the heart without any problem of acoustic window or signal attenuation. The multiplanar capability of CMR permit to generate images from any anatomical cardiac plane with high reproducibility and without the need for post-processing reconstruction. By this, CMR may provide accurate evaluation of tricuspid and sub-tricuspid apparatus morphology and function. Moreover, thorough tissue characterization capability, CMR allows detection of right ventricular disease often associated to isolated tricuspid regurgitation as right ventricular arrhythmogenic cardiomyopathy, pulmonary hypertension and congenital heart disease.

Morphological and Functional Assessment

CMR may visualize all the parts of tricuspid apparatus as leaflets, annulus, chordae tendineae, and papillary muscles throughout the entire cardiac cycle in similar way of echocardiography [4] but with a multiplanar approach by the acquisition of several "radial" slices centered on the tricuspid plane and passing through the cardiac apex (Figure 1).

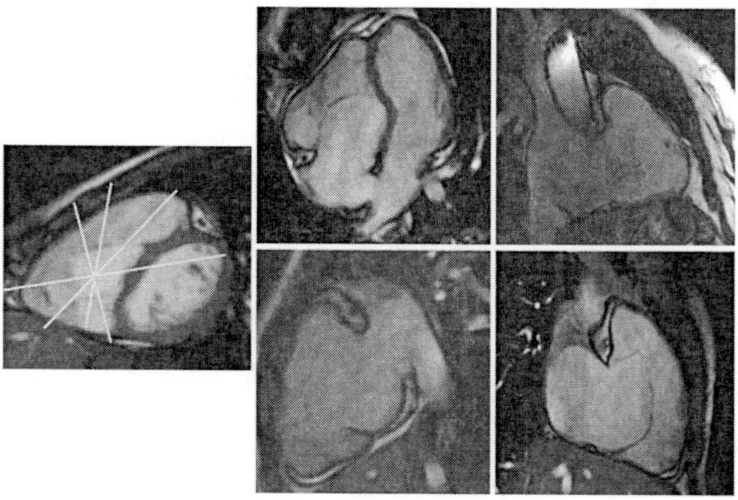

Figure 1. Example of radial acquisition of cine-SSFP images of cardiac magnetic resonance in a patient with Ebstein's anomaly.

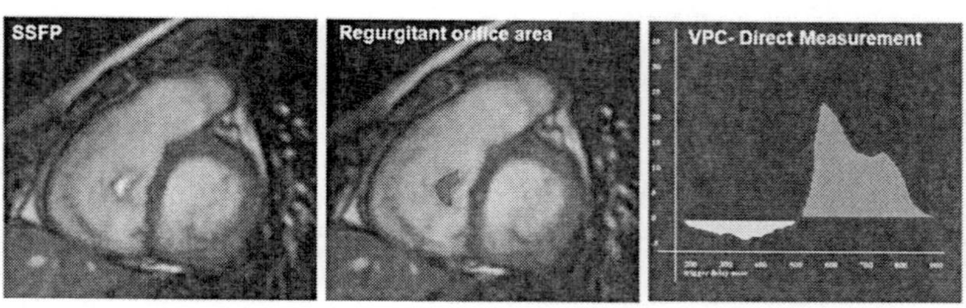

Figure 2. Quantification of regurgitant orifice area of tricuspid regurgitation by planimetric area contouring (left and middle panels) and through a direct measurement of regurgitant volume by Velocity Encodend Phase Contrast technique (right panel). In the right panel the regurgitant volume is measured as the integral of the negative part of the curve.

CMR is generally considered the gold standard imaging technique for the evaluation of ventricular volumes as well as for the evaluation of functional parameters as ejection fraction and the right and left stroke volumes. Moreover, CMR is a valuable imaging technique for the quantification of valvular regurgitant volume and regurgitant fraction. Steady state free precession (SSFP) and gradient echo cine pulse sequences can image regurgitating "jets" on the basis of loss of signal (signal void) of flow turbulence due to the dephasing of moving protons. SSFP, implemented to increase the contrast between myocardium and blood, is less sensitive for depicting flow disturbance and this causes an underestimation of a regurgitant jet. Gradient echo cine pulse sequences are more sensitive for the detection and sizing of regurgitant jets. With gradient echo sequences, the sensitivity for detecting regurgitation jets is a function of the echo time: the longer the echo time, the larger and more pronounced the regurgitant jet. Echo time should be appropriately set before the acquisition of the images in order to evaluate the regurgitant jets. CMR tends also to underestimate tricuspid regurgitating jet because of lower flow velocities than for mitral regurgitation. Then regurgitant jet evaluation is limited to just a qualitative assessment of tricuspid regurgitation. By the acquisition of short axis cine images at the atrioventricular plane, CMR provide direct planimetric measurement of the tricuspid regurgitant orifice (Figure 2).

Quantitative measurement of tricuspid valvular regurgitation by CMR is generally preferred to all these qualitative or semiquantitative approaches for evaluation of severity of tricuspid regurgitation. Velocity encoded phase contrast imaging (VPC) is a cine-CMR technique for directly quantifying flowing blood in vascular district [5]. The net through plane flow in measured in each cardiac phase by the multiplication of cross-sectional area and average velocities. A flow/time curve of the entire cardiac cycle is generated as in Figure 2: the instantaneous flow volume of each frame (y-axis) are plotted against the time of the cardiac cycle (x-axis). Using this technique, it is possible to obtain a direct measurement of anterograde flow in ascending aorta and pulmonary artery and to quantify the cardiac output, measured respectively as systemic flow (Qs) and pulmonary flow (Qp) and to evaluate the presence of cardiac shunts (Qp/Qs ratio > or < 1) [6]. The area under the forward part of the curve represents the total flow in systole through the valve and the area under the backward diastolic part, when present, is the retrograde regurgitating volume which may be directly measured. This approach may be also used to "directly" quantify tricuspid and mitral regurgitation.

However, this "direct method" of quantification is very robust and reproducible for pulmonary and aortic regurgitation but has several limitations for tricuspid and mitral valve. In fact, a correct acquisition plane is mandatory for a valid quantification of flow because measurement of flow is most precise if main direction of flow and through-plane flow encoding are orthogonal to the imaging plane. A > 15° angle deviation from the orthogonal plane is considered not tolerable producing an underestimation of the flow [7]. Moreover, 2D - VPC technique provides accurate estimation of flow velocities for laminar flow but underestimates turbulent flow. For mitral and tricuspid regurgitation, the direct measurement of regurgitation volume by VPC is less accurate and reproducible than for aortic and pulmonary valves, because of the base-to-apex ventricular shift during of atrioventricular plane during systole, for the complex morphology of the atrioventricular valves and for the turbulent flow inside the ventricles and atria.

Then, it is preferable to use an "indirect method" to calculate the tricuspid regurgitation volume: in absence of shunts (Qp/Qs = 1), the regurgitation volume of tricuspid valve is measured as the difference between the right ventricular stroke volume and the anterograde flow in pulmonary flow (corrected for any amount of pulmonary regurgitation) measured by the VPC technique [8].

For the assessment of right ventricular stroke volume, the established CMR method requires acquisition of a volumetric stack of electrocardiogram-gated short-axis images covering the entire left and right ventricular myocardium from atrioventricular planes to the apex.

For each short axis section, images are acquired in a time-sequence fashion defined as "cine"- imaging. Ventricular short axis images are acquired on parallel planes with a fixed slice thickness (usually 8 mm) and without a gap between each slice. Image analysis is performed by the manual or automatic tracking of the endocardial and epicardial contours of both ventricles in the end-diastole and end-systole phase. The areas within the endocardial and epicardial contours are measured in each slice and multiplied for thickness to obtain respectively the blood pool volume and the myocardial volume of the slice. Then, accordingly to the modified Simpson's rule, the ventricular volumes and myocardial volumes are obtained by the summation of respectively the blood pool volumes and myocardial volumes of each slice.

The stroke volume is measured in each ventricle by the subtraction of the end-systolic from the end-diastolic volumes and ejection fraction as the ratio, expressed in percentage, between stroke volume and end-diastolic volume.

Quantification of ventricular volumes and functional parameters with CMR may be also affected by artefacts in presence of arrhythmias as atrial fibrillation and frequent premature complexes. In these circumstances, the R-R variation may significantly limit the accuracy of volumes quantification not permitting the evaluation of SV.

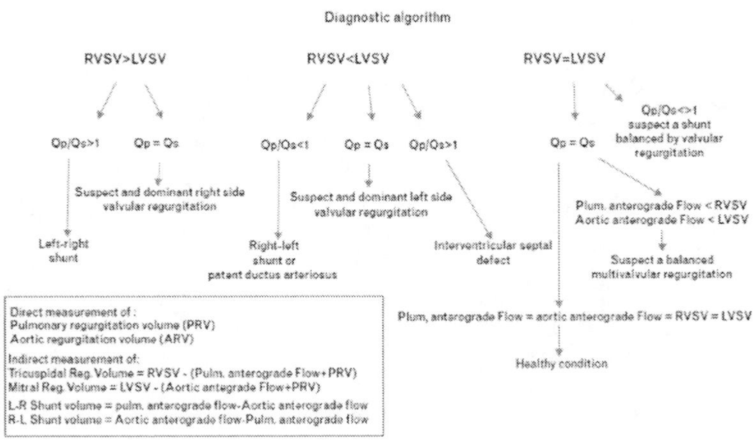

Figure 3. Diagnostic algorithm for diagnosis and quantification of cardiac valvular regurgitation and shunts (with permission from Aquaro et al., J Cardiovasc Med. 2015; 16(10): 663-70).

Despite this limit, the inter-study reproducibility for the quantification of ventricular volumes by CMR is higher than echocardiography, permitting to decrease from 55 to 93% the sample size of study population in clinical trials [9].

Moreover, the inter- and intra-observer reproducibility of CMR for the evaluation of ventricular functional parameters is very good, and in the clinical setting a discrepancy of > 5 ml of volumes or > 5 grams of ventricular mass is generally not tolerated [10].

Tricuspid regurgitation may also be part of a more complex condition in patient with congenital heart disease. In this setting, CMR with the combination of ventricular stroke volume measurement by cine-imaging and Qp/Qs measurement by VPC technique may provide an accurate valuation of cardiac physiology allowing quantification of shunt volumes and regurgitation volumes (Figure 3) and adequate surgical planning.

Finally, 4D-Flow is a promising CMR technique providing dynamic three-dimensional evaluation of both cine and flow velocity imaging in all the cardiac phase in a single acquisition. This technique might potentially permit direct contemporary quantification of cardiac function, volumes, valvular regurgitation volume and shunt volume without any limitation of flow direction and velocities (Figure 4).

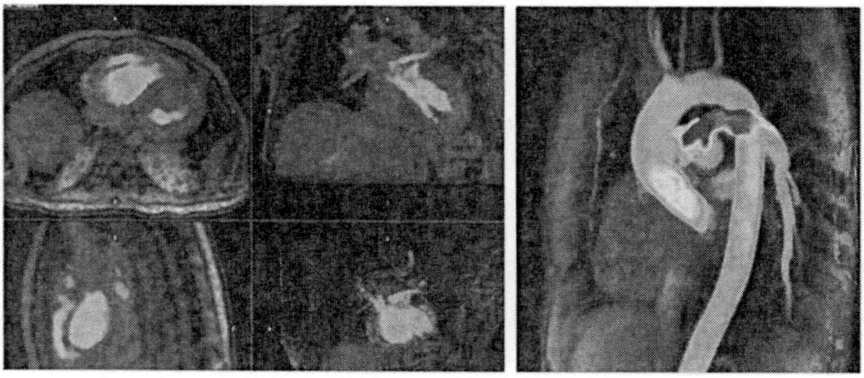

Figure 4. Examples of different reconstruction planes of new 4D-flow technique by CMR.

Myocardial Disease Assessment

CMR is also considered a valuable imaging technique for the evaluation of myocardial disease that may be associated to tricuspid regurgitation. Arrhythmogenic right ventricular cardiomyopathy is characterized by fibro-fatty replacement of right ventricular myocardium, associated to right ventricular regional wall motion abnormality and eventually to dilation and dysfunction. In this latter circumstance, a tricuspid annular dilation may produce a significant regurgitation. CMR may give an accurate evaluation of myocardial tissue abnormalities as fat infiltration and fibrosis in this condition and of regional and global wall motion abnormalities, providing a diagnosis of this cardiomyopathy. This is very relevant for the management of the patients because in this condition valvular surgical correction could not improve the outcome of the patients because of the high risk of cardiac arrhythmic death.

Functional tricuspid regurgitation may occur in presence of right ventricular overload in presence of conditions which may be unrecognized by echocardiography, as partial anomalous pulmonary venous connection or Ebstein Anomaly, or subclinical phase of pulmonary hypertension, In these cases, CMR may establish a definite diagnosis permitting and to plan the adequate therapy.

CMR is also a valuable technique for the characterization of cardiac tumors and masses involving tricuspid valve. However, tissue characterization of these masses by CMR is limited by the high mobility and by the reduced dimension (< 5 mm) [11].

CMR for Timing of Tricuspid Valve Surgery and for Outcomes Prediction

An accurate quantification of regurgitant volume may be very important for patient management. Uretsky and colleagues demonstrated that in patients with mitral regurgitation, CMR assessment of severity by the measurement of regurgitation volume is more accurate than echocardiography to predict the amount of post-surgical reverse remodeling [12]. This data may be also valid for tricuspid regurgitation. In fact, in an ideal model of valvular regurgitation, the regurgitant volume may predict the reverse remodeling after valvular correction because this volume participates to end-diastolic volume and to ventricular overload. In a case of severe right ventricular dilation with great tricuspid regurgitant volume one may aspect a significant reduction of ventricular end-diastolic volume after surgery, which instead may not be found in the opposite condition of severe ventricular dilation but with low regurgitant volume.

In a cohort of 75 patients undergoing tricuspid valve correction for severe regurgitation, Park and colleagues demonstrated that volumetric quantification of RV end-systolic volume index and RV ejection fraction by CMR are important predictor of all-cause and cardiac mortality [13].

In a small population study Kim and colleagues confirmed the reliability of CMR to assess volume changes of right ventricle after surgical correction of tricuspid regurgitation and demonstrated that right ventricular volume assessed by this technique may be effective to choose the optimal timing for surgical correction [14].

Cardiac Computed Tomography

Multislice CT provides more detailed and reproducible geometric measurements and 4-dimensional delineation of the right heart (Figure 5).

Compared with the mitral valve, which can be optimally evaluated in most routine coronary CT angiography studies, visualization of the right atrioventricular junction in detail can be challenging. Clear depiction of this region requires homogeneous enhancement of the structures around the tricuspid valve annulus.

The normal morphology of the Tricuspid Valve can be clearly depicted by CT even if it has an elliptical shape and appears nonplanar, with the posteroseptal portion “lowest” (toward the apex) [15]. In severe functional tricuspid regurgitation (FTR), the annulus becomes planar and flat [8] (Figure 6).

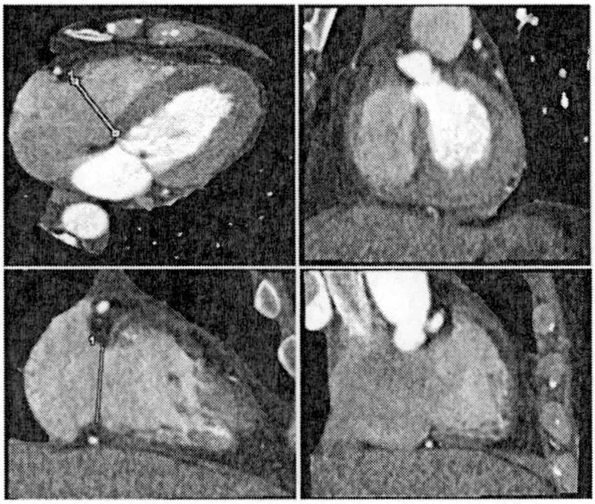

Figure 5. Reconstructed CT-images of tricuspid valve in different planes.

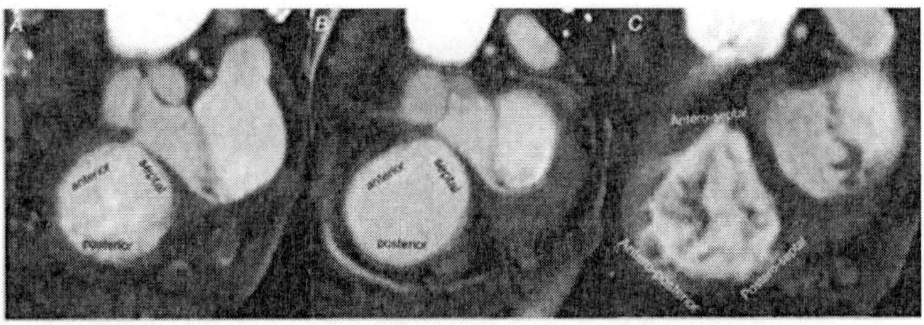

Figure 6. MPR CT images showing the morphology of the tricuspid annulus (TA) in patient with functional regurgitation during diastole (A) and systole (B) defining the tricuspid TA and localization of the three commissures (C).

During the cardiac cycle, the annulus area changes by approximately one-third, with the diameter changing by one-fifth [16, 17]. ECG-gated CT reveals this unique tricuspid morphology of the annulus, along with its temporal changes in different phases of the cardiac cycle (Figure 7).

In functional tricuspid regurgitation (FTR), the tricuspid annulus becomes more planar, dilating primarily in the septal-lateral direction, thus producing a more circular shape compared with the elliptical shape in healthy subjects. Dilatation of the annulus involves the mural side of the annulus, not the septal side. The critical diameter of the annulus for FTR is around 27 mm/m^2 [18]. CT may further facilitate the decision regarding the type of surgery by enabling accurate characterization of leaflet tethering [19].

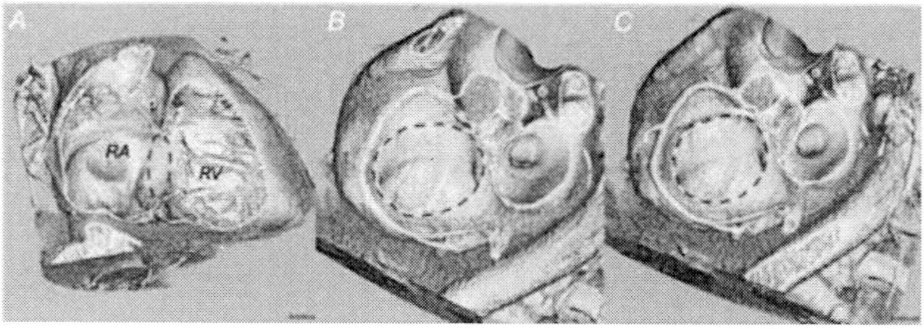

Figure 7. 3D-cut plane endoscopy CT images showing the localization of the RCA and the TA position at the atrioventricular groove which permit the accurate measurements of diameters and perimeter and its anatomical relationship with hinge line of leaflets through the long axis of the right heart (A); the course of the RCA into the atrioventricular groove encircling the tricuspid annulus (red dotted ellipse) during systole (B) and diastole (C).

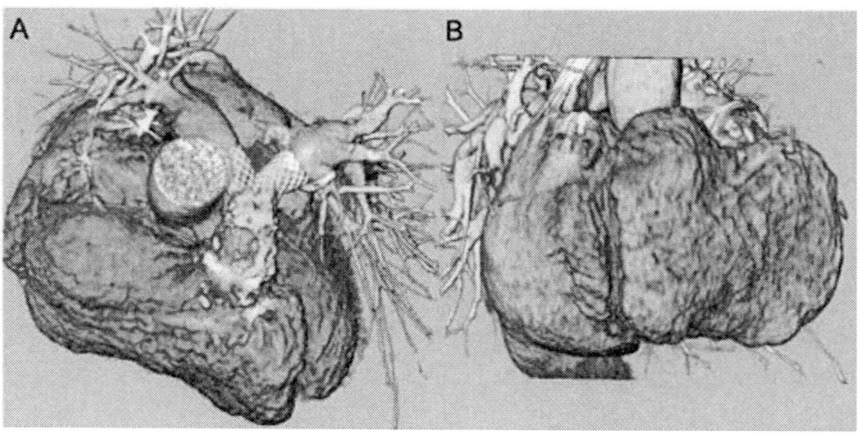

Figure 8. CCT 3D-Volume Rendering images of a patient with right chambers dilation in corrected Tetralogy of Fallot with calcified pulmonary conduit and stents of the main pulmonary branches, tricuspid valvuloplasty and pacemaker leads.

Primary malformations of the Tricuspid Valve (TV) are rare anomalies, with the Ebstein anomaly the most common. In contrast, secondary tricuspid dysfunction is a common associated finding in adult congenital heart disease (CHD), typically related to chronic right ventricle (RV) volume overloading (i.e., or corrected Tetralogy of Fallot). Functional tricuspid regurgitation is also common in the systemic RV because of pressure and volume overload (i.e., corrected transposition of the great arteries) [20].

Cardiac CT generates volumes with submillimetric, isotropic voxels, which permit to analyze cardiac chambers and vascular structures with multi-planar (MPR), volume rendering (3D-VR) and in motion reconstructions, useful in planning surgical and interventional procedures (Figure 8).

The CT scan data set has to include TV, all the heart and IVC or SVC. The mixed tail of the contrast bolus can provide homogeneous visualization of SVC. In case of tricuspid insufficiency, during the breath-hold necessary for the CT scan, the IVC is retrogradely opacified in relation to the inverted flux towards the hepatic veins.

Most ECG gated or triggered cardiac CTA techniques modified for the right heart examination (i.e., 50% contrast agent and saline chase in routine coronary CTA) can provide good-quality motion-free images of the RV outlet and trabeculated portions. However, the quality may not be high enough to show the details of RV inlet [21]. This is mainly because of inhomogeneous enhancement of the right atrium and artifacts arising from high-attenuation superior vena cava contrast enhancement when mixed with unenhanced blood of the inferior vena cava. The right atrial artifacts may be decreased when injections are performed through the femoral vein. The best results, however, may be obtained with simultaneous injection of contrast agent in both femoral and antecubital veins. Despite this consideration, most of the studies evaluating the role of CT for tricuspid valve morphologic assessment use a triphasic protocol of contrast agent infusion in the antecubital vein (60–80ml contrast with a flow-rate of 5.0–6.0ml/s, followed by a 20ml mixture of 1:1 contrast and saline and 25ml of saline) and the scanning is started at peak enhancement of left ventricle.

A retrospective CCT acquisition allow the possibility to reconstruct R-R interval sub-series identifying the diastolic and systolic phases. This kind of acquisition permits to evaluate and quantify the left but also right chambers functional parameters. CCT provides accurate and reproducible LV and RV volume parameters compared with MR, and can be considered as a reliable alternative for patients who are not suitable to undergo MR [22]. In patients with atrial fibrillation the limited temporal resolution of cardiac-CT may be cause of underestimation of right ventricular function and volumes. In the majority of cases, however, the tricuspid valve functional anatomy can be seen in its entire extent.

One advantage of CT is that it can show the extent of calcifications in this region. Degenerative calcium deposition in the TV annulus is relatively rare compared with the mitral annulus, likely because of an incomplete fibrous ring on the right side. Reported calcifications are usually secondary to diffuse cardiac calcinosis in chronic dialysis patients and in patients with inflammatory processes, such as rheumatic heart disease [23].

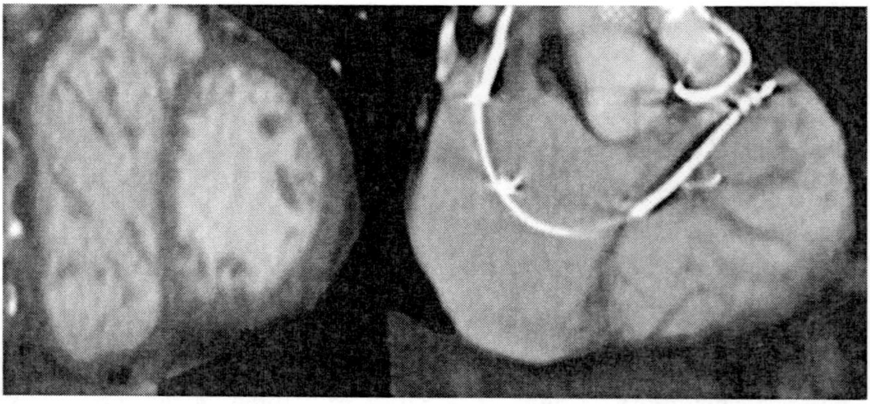

Figure 9. CCT Multi-Planar Reformatted images of corrected Tetralogy of Fallot showing dilated right chambers and "D-shaped" interventricular septum (two-chambers view, left side). The right ventricular lead moves through the tricuspid valve with the catheter tip adjacent to the pulmonary outflow tract (two-chambers long axis view, right side).

Is also possible to identify pericardial calcifications related to pericarditis and show the relation to the right ventricle and its relation with the sternum.

CT also enables evaluation of tricuspid valve annuloplasty ring dislodgement and helps identify inappropriate position of the ventricular pacemaker lead at the tricuspid level and related complications (Figure 9).

The role of CT imaging to help with patient screening and procedural planning of transcatheter tricuspid valve interventions is less well established than for the planning of mitral and aortic interventions. For planning transcatheter interventions of tricuspid regurgitation, of particular importance are the structures that have a spatial relationship with the tricuspid valve annulus such as the right coronary artery. In a population of 250 patients Van Rosendae and colleagues demonstrated the effectiveness of Computed tomography to characterize the spatial relationship between the right coronary artery and the tricuspid valve annulus which is pivotal for preventing coronary artery impingement during percutaneous tricuspid valve annulus procedures [8]. CT provides also geometrical information of the right ventricle relative to the tricuspid valve annulus facilitating the implantation of a spacer system. Finally, CT is a useful technique to depict the inferior vena cava and to achieve the sizing of caval valves in the planning of heterotopic implantation.

The main limits of CCT are represented by ionized radiations that, even if significantly reduced [24], limit its use over time and the administration of iodinated contrast media with renal function hazard; moreover, it does not allow the quantification of vascular flows.

Cardiopulmonary Exercise Test

Cardiopulmonary exercise testing (CPET) provides assessment of the integrative exercise responses involving the pulmonary, cardiovascular, hematopoietic, neuropsychological, and skeletal muscle systems, which are not fully reflected through the simple "sum" of the measurement of individual organ system function [25]. Bridging between mitochondria and outer atmosphere is provided by muscular, cardiovascular and respiratory systems.

CPET is a non-invasive, dynamic physiological test allowing assessment of both submaximal and peak exercise responses, providing physicians with relevant information for clinical decision making. The added value of the CPET lies on the fact that resting pulmonary and cardiac function testing (e.g., spirometry and echocardiography) cannot reliably predict exercise performance and functional capacity.

CPET Imaging

CPET imaging results from the combination of echocardiogram and CPET performed at the same time. CPET imaging has been widely tested in the evaluation of heart failure and in patients eligible for a heart transplantation. Combined CPET and exercise stress echocardiography technique proved to be feasible, providing a non-invasive evaluation of the hemodynamic and metabolic responses to exercise. Since multiple mechanisms are held responsible for the limited exercise capacity of patients with HF, the refinement of hemodynamic behavior during effort provided by echocardiography allows a better characterization of the primary cause of reduced exercise tolerance [26]. Furthermore, CPET imaging provided new insight on the role of right ventricle – pulmonary vasculature (RV-PV) uncoupling in intolerance to exercise. In 2014 CPET imaging has been used to study a population of 136 patients with different cardiovascular diseases suffering from intolerance to exercise [27]. In that case multivariate-analysis shown that the main determinants of a premature flattening of VO2/WR function are exercise systolic pulmonary artery pressure and tricuspidal annular plane systolic excursion. Dynamic evaluation of RV function during exercise indeed enables the assessment of RV contractile reserve and helps unmask subclinical dysfunction in different cardiovascular diseases, as in the case of pulmonary hypertension [28] or mitral stenosis [29] and, theoretically, in primitive diseases of the tricuspid valve. The combined tests are extremely useful in patients with "intermediate range" cardiovascular diseases, particularly when symptoms are out of proportion to resting hemodynamics.

References

[1] Nath, J., Foster, E. & Heidenreich, P. A. (2004). Impact of Tricuspid Regurgitation on Long-Term Survival. *J Am Coll Cardiol*, *43*, 405–409.

[2] Rogers, J. H. & Bolling, S. F. (2009). The tricuspid valve: Current perspective and evolving management of tricuspid regurgitation. *Circulation*, *119*, 2718–2725.

[3] Faletra, F. F., Leo, L. A., Paiocchi, V. L., Schlossbauer, S. A., Borruso, M. G., Pedrazzini, G., Moccetti, T. & Ho, S. Y. (2018). Imaging-based tricuspid valve anatomy by computed tomography, magnetic resonance imaging, two and three-dimensional echocardiography: correlation with anatomic specimen. *Eur Heart J - Cardiovasc Imaging*, *20*, 1–13.

[4] Cawley, P. J., Maki, J. H. & Otto, C. M. (2009). Cardiovascular magnetic resonance imaging for valvular heart disease: technique and validation. *Circulation*, *119*, 468–478.

[5] Nayler, G., Firmin, D., Longmore, D. & others. (1986). Blood flow imaging by cine magnetic resonance. *J Comput Assist Tomogr*, *10*, 715–722.

[6] Aquaro, G. D., Barison, A., Todiere, G., Festa, P., Ait-Ali, L., Lombardi, M., Di Bella, G. & others. (2015). Cardiac magnetic resonance 'virtual catheterization' for the quantification of valvular regurgitations and cardiac shunt. *J Cardiovasc Med*, *16*, 663.

[7] Yang, G. Z., Burger, P., Kilner, P. J., Karwatowski, S. P. & Firmin, D. N. (1996). Dynamic range extension of cine velocity measurements using motion registered spatiotemporal phase unwrapping. *J Magn Reson Imaging*, *6*, 495–502.

[8] van Rosendael, P. J., Kamperidis, V., Kong, W. K. F., van Rosendael, A. R., van der Kley, F., Ajmone Marsan, N., Delgado, V. & Bax, J. J. (2017). Computed tomography for planning transcatheter tricuspid valve therapy. *Eur Heart J*, *38*, 665–674.

[9] Gandy, S. J., Waugh, S. A., Nicholas, R. S., Simpson, H. J., Milne, W. & Houston, J. G. (2008). Comparison of the reproducibility of

quantitative cardiac left ventricular assessments in healthy volunteers using different MRI scanners: a multicenter simulation. *J Magn Reson Imaging JMRI*, *28*, 359–365.

[10] Maceira, A. M., Prasad, S. K., Khan, M. & Pennell, D. J. (2006). Normalized left ventricular systolic and diastolic function by steady state free precession cardiovascular magnetic resonance. *J Cardiovasc Magn Reson Off J Soc Cardiovasc Magn Reson*, *8*, 417–426.

[11] Bianco, F., Bucciarelli, V., Todiere, G., Barison, A., Festa, P., Ait-Ali, L., Gallina, S., De Caterina, R. & Aquaro, G. D. (2017). Cardiac tumors: role of magnetic resonance imaging. *G Ital Cardiol*, 2006, *18*, 286–294.

[12] Uretsky, S., Argulian, E., Narula, J. & Wolff, S. D. (2018). Use of Cardiac Magnetic Resonance Imaging in Assessing Mitral Regurgitation: Current Evidence. *J Am Coll Cardiol*, *71*, 547–563.

[13] Park, J. B., Kim, H. K., Jung, J. H., et al. (2016). Prognostic Value of Cardiac MR Imaging for Preoperative Assessment of Patients with Severe Functional Tricuspid Regurgitation. *Radiology*, *280*, 723–734.

[14] Kim, H. K., Kim, Y. J., Park, E. A., et al. (2010). Assessment of haemodynamic effects of surgical correction for severe functional tricuspid regurgitation: cardiac magnetic resonance imaging study. *Eur Heart J*, *31*, 1520–1528.

[15] Fukuda, S. (2006). Three-Dimensional Geometry of the Tricuspid Annulus in Healthy Subjects and in Patients With Functional Tricuspid Regurgitation: A Real-Time, 3-Dimensional Echocardiographic Study. *Circulation*, *114*, I–492–I–498.

[16] Tei, C., Pilgrim, J. P., Shah, P. M., Ormiston, J. A. & Wong, M. (1982). The tricuspid valve annulus: study of size and motion in normal subjects and in patients with tricuspid regurgitation. *Circulation*, *66*, 665–671.

[17] Ton-Nu, T. T., Levine, R. A., Handschumacher, M. D., Dorer, D. J., Yosefy, C., Fan, D., Hua, L., Jiang, L. & Hung, J. (2006). Geometric determinants of functional tricuspid regurgitation: insights from 3-dimensional echocardiography. *Circulation*, *114*, 143–149.

[18] Ubago, J. L., Figueroa, A., Ochoteco, A., Colman, T., Duran, R. M. & Duran, C. G. (1983). Analysis of the amount of tricuspid valve anular dilatation required to produce functional tricuspid regurgitation. *Am J Cardiol*, *52*, 155–158.

[19] van Rosendael, P. J., Joyce, E., Katsanos, S., Debonnaire, P., Kamperidis, V., van der Kley, F., Schalij, M. J., Bax, J. J., Ajmone, Marsan N. & Delgado, V. (2016). Tricuspid valve remodelling in functional tricuspid regurgitation: multidetector row computed tomography insights. *Eur Heart J Cardiovasc Imaging*, *17*, 96–105.

[20] Giamberti, A., Chessa, M., Ballotta, A., Varrica, A., Agnetti, A., Frigiola, A. & Ranucci, M. (2011). Functional tricuspid valve regurgitation in adults with congenital heart disease: an emerging problem. *J Heart Valve Dis*, *20*, 565–570.

[21] Saremi, F., Ho, S. Y., Cabrera, J. A. & Sánchez-Quintana, D. (2013). Right ventricular outflow tract imaging with CT and MRI: Part 1, Morphology. *AJR Am J Roentgenol*, *200*, W39-50.

[22] Maffei, E., Messalli, G., Martini, C., et al. (2012). Left and right ventricle assessment with Cardiac CT: validation study vs. Cardiac MR. *Eur Radiol*, *22*, 1041–1049.

[23] Gould, L., Zahir, M., DeMartino, A., Gomprecht, R. F. & Hayt, D. (1971). Extensive calcification of the tricuspid valve in rheumatic heart disease. *Angiology*, *22*, 529–532.

[24] Maffei, E., Martini, C., De Crescenzo, S., et al. (2010). Low dose CT of the heart: a quantum leap into a new era of cardiovascular imaging. *Radiol Med (Torino)*, *115*, 1179–1207.

[25] Guazzi, M., Bandera, F., Ozemek, C., Systrom, D. & Arena, R. (2017). Cardiopulmonary Exercise Testing: What Is its Value? *J Am Coll Cardiol*, *70*, 1618–1636.

[26] Shimiaie, J., Sherez, J., Aviram, G., et al. (2015). Determinants of Effort Intolerance in Patients With Heart Failure: Combined Echocardiography and Cardiopulmonary Stress Protocol. *JACC Heart Fail*, *3*, 803–814.

[27] Bandera, F., Generati, G., Pellegrino, M., Donghi, V., Alfonzetti, E., Gaeta, M., Villani, S. & Guazzi, M. (2014). Role of right ventricle

and dynamic pulmonary hypertension on determining ΔVO2/ΔWork Rate flattening: insights from cardiopulmonary exercise test combined with exercise echocardiography. *Circ Heart Fail*, *7*, 782–790.

[28] Guo, D. C., Li, Y. D., Yang, Y. H., Zhu, W. W., Sun, L. L., Jiang, W., Ye, X. G., Cai, Q. Z. & Lu, X. Z. (2019). Influence of impaired right ventricular contractile reserve on exercise capacity in patients with precapillary pulmonary hypertension: A study with exercise stress echocardiography. *Echocardiogr Mt Kisco N*, *36*, 671–677.

[29] Laufer-Perl, M., Gura, Y., Shimiaie, J., et al. (2017). Mechanisms of Effort Intolerance in Patients With Rheumatic Mitral Stenosis: Combined Echocardiography and Cardiopulmonary Stress Protocol. *JACC Cardiovasc Imaging*, *10*, 622–633.

In: The Rediscovered Tricuspid Valve
Editor: Giacomo Bianchi
ISBN: 978-1-53616-098-7

Chapter 6

FUNCTIONAL DISEASE: TRICUSPID VALVE IN LEFT-SIDED HEART DISEASE

Giovanni Benfari[1], MD, Andrea Rossi[1], MD and Francesco Grigioni[2,*], MD, PhD
[1]Section of Cardiolgy, Department of Medicine, University of Verona, Verona, Italy
[2]Associate Professor of Cardiology, Head of Cardiology Unit, University Campus Biomedico of Rome, Rome, Italy

ABSTRACT

Functional tricuspid regurgitation is the most frequent right-side valvular disease encountered in routine practice. The prevalence of significant functional tricuspid regurgitation increases from <3% in the general population to >30% in patients with left ventricular dysfunction. Mitral valve disease and atrial fibrillation are other important clinical contexts of functional tricuspid regurgitation. Significant tricuspid regurgitation can also be present at the time of left-sided valve surgery, or develop over time after cardiac surgery. A deep and integrated knowledge of pathophysiology, clinical presentation and natural history of functional

* Corresponding Author's E-mail: f.grigioni@unicampus.it.

tricuspid regurgitation can help planning the appropriate medical or surgical intervention.

Keywords: functional disease, left-sided heart disease, tricuspid valve

EPIDEMIOLOGY AND CLINICAL SETTING

Functional tricuspid regurgitation (fTR) is the most frequent tricuspid valve disease in Western countries [1]. The most common mechanism which leads to functional tricuspid regurgitation is right ventricular dilation and dysfunction from left-sided heart disease, as in cases of significant mitral valve disease. Dilated cardiomyopathy and pulmonary hypertension are less frequent causes of tricuspid regurgitation. Other relevant conditions are atrial fibrillation and implanted cardiac devices with leads across the tricuspid valve.

In the general population, the prevalence of moderate to severe tricuspid regurgitation varies from 1.8% in the Atherosclerotic Risk in Communities population [2] to 2.7% in the OxVALVE Population Cohort Study [3]. In the setting of left-sided heart disease, the prevalence of functional tricuspid regurgitation became particularly high. Among patients with significant left ventricular dysfunction (ejection fraction ≤ 35%) the prevalence of moderate to severe tricuspid regurgitation varies from 30% in a cohort of 3943 patients [4] to 34.5% in a different cohort of 1436 patients [5]. Such relevant burden of tricuspid regurgitation has only recently gained attention, since this valve disease has long been considered as a surrogate of a primary condition, often affecting the left ventricle or left-sided valves [6]. Moreover, tricuspid regurgitation has been historically associated with left heart failure through elevated left-sided filling pressure and subsequent pulmonary artery hypertension. Pulmonary hypertension is a common complication of left heart failure [7], with a prevalence in heart failure with reduced ejection fraction (HFrEF) that ranges from 35% [8] to 47.5% [9]. However, not all patients with pulmonary hypertension develop significant tricuspid regurgitation, meaning that pulmonary hypertension and tricuspid regurgitation are not invariably linked [10].

In patients with mitral valve disease, the prevalence of functional tricuspid regurgitation is high as well: 30% of patients with degenerative mitral regurgitation have tricuspid regurgitation at the time of mitral valve surgery, and up to one-third of patients with significant mitral stenosis have moderate to severe tricuspid regurgitation [11]. Among patients with ischemic mitral regurgitation, 30% of those who underwent revascularization and mitral valve surgery has tricuspid regurgitation [12].

Functional tricuspid regurgitation is particularly frequent among patients with mitral valve prolapse. The mitral valve prolapse has a prevalence in the Framingham Heart Study of 2.5% in men and 7.6% in women [13] and, currently, mitral valve prolapse is the most common disorder leading to mitral valve surgery. In patients with mitral valve prolapse, functional tricuspid regurgitation prevalence and degree mostly depends to the stage of the mitral disease, being higher in the late stages, when tricuspid disease reflects the presence and severity of right ventricle failure; a moderate to severe tricuspid regurgitation is present in up to 16% of the patients referred for surgery for mitral valve prolapse [14], a prevalence higher compared to 8% in patients referred to surgery for severe mitral regurgitation of all etiologies [15]. Although secondary tricuspid regurgitation is the most involved alteration in this setting, primary tricuspid regurgitation has to be mentioned, in particular tricuspid valve prolapse. Prevalence of tricuspid valve prolapse in patients without other valvular disease is extremely rare. On the contrary, association of tricuspid and mitral valve prolapse is relevant, who seems to share the same tissue alterations, with a prevalence close to 54% of patients [16]. Notably, concomitant mitral and tricuspid valve prolapse often occurs in patients with Marfan syndrome and other connective tissue diseases (Ehlers Danlos Syndrome, osteogenesis imperfecta, etc.) [17].

Functional tricuspid regurgitation can also occur after left-sided valve surgery, in patients without pre-existing significant tricuspid regurgitation. New-development of significant tricuspid regurgitation late after left heart valve procedure varies between 9% and 49% of cases [18], whereas the worsening of tricuspid regurgitation severity grade, with respect to preoperative status, is reported in about 14% of patients during a mean 4 years follow-up after isolated mitral valve repair due to mitral prolapse [11].

PATHOPHYSIOLOGY

Functional tricuspid regurgitation is mainly the result of annular dilation and right ventricular enlargement, which are often consequences of left heart failure from myocardial or valvular causes [11]. The mechanisms behind the right ventricular alteration are complex and heterogeneous. Indeed, patients with non-ischemic and ischemic cardiomyopathy or left valvular heart disease, could present with increased left ventricular preload and/or afterload, decreased myocardial function, dilation of the cardiac chambers and elevated atrial pressures, which lead to right ventricular volume and pressure overload, with or without elevation in pulmonary artery pressure. The occurrence of functional TR reflects these underlying hemodynamic changes [19].

Right Ventricular Dilation and Dysfunction

Whatever the cause of LV dysfunction, the pathophysiologic pathway from left-sided heart disease to functional tricuspid regurgitation begins with a rise in left atrial pressure, which is transmitted through the lungs as pulmonary hypertension, which in turn causes right ventricular dilation. The relatively thin muscular mass of the right ventricular free wall makes it more load sensitive so that the pressure overload brought by pulmonary hypertension results in early right ventricular enlargement and systolic functional impairment [20]. The initial dilatation of the right ventricle causes the tricuspid annulus to dilate. In this early stage, tricuspid regurgitation may still be absent [21]. With progressive right ventricular and tricuspid annulus dilation, the right ventricle becomes distorted with consequent displacement of the papillary muscle attached to the right ventricular free wall and increasing in the tenting volume.

Moreover, with tricuspid annulus dilation, the normal papillary muscle-to-leaflet and annulus relationship is further altered, and the low points of the annulus may be stretched away from the papillary muscles, thereby increasing tethering. At this stage, leaflet coaptation fails and functional tricuspid regurgitation occurs [22]. Tricuspid regurgitation itself contributes to pressure and volume overload, further right ventricular enlargement, thereby increasing the tethering of the tricuspid valve leaflets and, as a result, the severity of TR itself.

Notably, once the tricuspid valve is dilated, its size cannot spontaneously return to normal, and it may continue to dilate further [11]. The right ventricular remodeling could be partly reversible, especially in the case of left-sided valvular heart disease and their correction [12], but right ventricular dysfunction may be irreversible.

So, both the development of tethering of the tricuspid valve leaflets and tricuspid valve annular dilatation are related to changes in right ventricular size and geometry. Interestingly, Fukuda et al. observed that left ventricular dysfunction impacted leaflet tethering but not on the annulus; however, tethering of the tricuspid valve leaflets is sufficient to cause tricuspid regurgitation even in the absence of significant tricuspid annular dilatation [23]. On the contrary, the dilatation of tricuspid annulus has been supposed to be more closely related to right atrial enlargement in patients with chronic atrial fibrillation than to right ventricular remodeling secondary to left-sided heart disease [24]. However, in patients with chronic left heart failure, right atrial volume was observed to increase with worsening left ventricular systolic and diastolic dysfunction [25].

Pulmonary Hypertension

Among stable heart failure with reduced ejection fraction outpatients, pulmonary hypertension is common and is associated with disease severity and survival [26]. It is closely related to diastolic dysfunction and severity of functional mitral regurgitation but not independently to the degree of left ventricular systolic dysfunction [7, 27]. Pulmonary hypertension from any cause has been associated with the development of functional tricuspid regurgitation through the pathway explained above. However, it is not a necessary prerequisite. Mutlak et al. observed that pulmonary hypertension does not invariably lead to tricuspid regurgitation [28]. In 2139 subjects with either mild, moderate, or severe elevations in pulmonary artery systolic pressure, an increasing pulmonary pressure level was independently associated with higher degrees of tricuspid regurgitation (odds ratio, 2.26 per 10 mmHg increase). However, many patients with high pulmonary pressure level had only mild tricuspid regurgitation. Moreover, other concomitant factors, such as atrial fibrillation, pacemaker leads, and right heart enlargement, were also importantly associated with tricuspid regurgitation severity. According to the authors, the cause of functional tricuspid regurgitation in pulmonary hypertension patients is only partially related to an increase in the trans-tricuspid pressure gradient, with remodeling of the right heart in response to elevated pulmonary artery systolic pressure as the major mechanism responsible for functional tricuspid regurgitation [29].

Fukuda et al. observed septal leaflet tethering in patients with functional tricuspid regurgitation and normal pulmonary artery pressure; a hypokinetic, dyskinetic, or dilated septum could lead to a tethering effect on the tricuspid valve, because of the right ventricle's septal wall that is the area of origin of the papillary muscles to the septal leaflet of the tricuspid valve, causing functional tricuspid regurgitation [23].

Moreover, the decrease of the pulmonary artery systolic pressure after mitral valve surgery does not always eliminate tricuspid regurgitation, or tricuspid regurgitation often develops years after surgery [12]. Neither it is proven that tricuspid regurgitation correction in the setting of pulmonary hypertension alters the natural course of right ventricular dilation and development of chronic right heart dysfunction [29].

Mitral Valve Prolapse

In functional tricuspid regurgitation related to mitral valve prolapse, the presence of tricuspid regurgitation is not to attribute to mitral disease per se, but has a complex and multifactorial pathogenesis. Two are the most critical mechanism involved in the pathophysiological process [30, 31]: leaflet tethering and tricuspid annular dilatation. Mitral regurgitation, due to blood pumped back into the left atrium, induces an increase in left atrial pressure, which progressively leads to pulmonary hypertension, right ventricular dysfunction, and enlargement causing an apical displacement of subvalvular structures, which results in tricuspid regurgitation [32].

Furthermore, mitral regurgitation due to mitral valve prolapse induces left atrial enlargement through increased left atrial pressure. Left atrial remodeling is associated with atrial fibrillation and subsequent tricuspid annular dilatation, the latter being a substratum for tricuspid regurgitation development [33].

The degree to which each of these two factors affects tricuspid regurgitation development is still controversial [31].

Left Ventricular-Right Ventricular Interdependence and Biventricular Failure

Left and right ventricular interdependence play an essential role in right ventricular function. In addition to a shared interventricular septum with helical fibers, which are not contained in the right ventricle free wall but in the septum [34], there is continuity between the muscle fibers of the two ventricles, resulting in a mechanical union whereby left ventricular contraction augments right ventricular free wall contraction. Experimental models have shown that 20% to 40% of right ventricular systolic pressure and volume outflow results from left ventricular contraction [35, 36]. Buckberg et al. noted that right ventricular failure does not occur after elimination of all right ventricular free wall muscle function after its exclusion by electrocautery, or its replacement by a plastic patch, but after embolization of the right coronary septal vessels, implying that the interventricular septum is the "right ventricular lion" [37]. Besides, the left and right ventricle may share a common biochemical milieu. Therefore, it could be postulated that surgical and/or medical treatment of the left-sided abnormality, which is the primary lesion, will result in secondary improvement of functional tricuspid regurgitation. However, although improvement in functional tricuspid regurgitation does occur, this is not invariably the case.

In patients with ischemic, non-ischemic, and valvular cardiomyopathy with left ventricular dysfunction, the presence of dilated left ventricles or increased left ventricular end-diastolic pressure lead to septal bowing, causing a wall motion disorder so that the septum results dyskinetic or hypokinetic. In these cases, the right ventricular free wall could be unable to compensate the septal dysfunction, and right ventricular failure will result because of impaired right ventricular filling, limited right ventricular contractile performance, and overload brought by pulmonary hypertension [37, 38].

Tricuspid Regurgitation after Left Heart Valve Procedure

The development or progression of functional tricuspid regurgitation late after left heart valve procedure represent a consequence of geometric alterations of the right ventricle. It has been described how in aortic stenosis patients, after aortic valve replacement, left ventricular hypertrophy decreases, but the degree of diffuse interstitial myocardial fibrosis remains unchanged [39]. Diffuse myocardial fibrosis is linked with diastolic dysfunction and elevated LV end-diastolic pressures, promoting post-capillary pulmonary hypertension [18]. Pulmonary hypertension causes right ventricular pressure overload, right ventricular dilation, distortion of the tricuspid valvular apparatus, and finally, significant tricuspid regurgitation. This pathogenetic process is supported by greater left atrial dilation and higher pulmonary pressure level in patients with severe tricuspid regurgitation [18].

Clinical Presentation

Patients with significant functional tricuspid regurgitation may remain asymptomatic, despite impaired right ventricular function [40]. Usually, symptoms related to concomitant left-sided valvular heart disease. Asthenia, fatigue and reduced exercise capacity may occur as a result of low cardiac output, whereas upper abdominal pain, ascites, and peripheral lower limb edema may accompany hepatic congestion due to elevated right atrial pressure.

Usually, isolated tricuspid regurgitation is clinically silent, and it is diagnosed at the time of echocardiographic evaluation of left-sided heart disease or evaluation of right heart failure. In advanced tricuspid regurgitation, signs and symptoms of right heart failure (systolic jugular distension, pulsatile hepatomegaly, and peripheral edema, signs on auscultation, right bundle branch block and atrial fibrillation on electrocardiogram, cardiomegaly on chest X-ray) don't differ from those of chronic right heart failure from other causes [21]. On auscultation, a soft pansystolic murmur at the lower sternal border and xiphoid process can be heard, caused by turbulent flow through the incompetent tricuspid valve into the right atrium, typically increasing in intensity during inspiration. However, these signs are non-specific and may be difficult to identify until relevant tricuspid regurgitation occurs. When mitral regurgitation coexists, the murmur of mitral regurgitation is a mid-frequency, rectangular, taking up all of the systole. Also, a third heart sound gallop in diastole could be heard in patients with heart failure, caused by deceleration of hematic flow from left atrium to the right ventricle [41].

Progression and Prognosis

Uncorrected severe tricuspid regurgitation, is considered a self-perpetuating disease, with patients needing increasing amounts of diuretics and frequently developing liver dysfunction. In left-sided heart disease secondary to mitral valve prolapse without left or right dysfunction, increased pulmonary artery pressure level and permanent atrial fibrillation are the most powerful risk factors for tricuspid regurgitation progression [31].

In patients with functional tricuspid regurgitation related to left-sided heart disease, both decreased left the ventricular systolic function, and elevated pulmonary artery pressure are well-known markers of poor survival [42, 43]. Nevertheless, functional tricuspid regurgitation seems to have a prognostic value per se that is proportional to its severity, even after adjustment for left ventricular function and systolic pulmonary artery pressure [40]. Topilsky et al. observed that the threshold of tricuspid regurgitation associated with excess mortality and excess event-rates was ERO $\geq$ 0.4 cm^2 [44]. Therefore, in this context, significant functional tricuspid regurgitation should be considered an additional and incremental marker of outcome. However, it remains unresolved whether functional tricuspid regurgitation is itself independently associated to mortality, and deserves a specific treatment, or it is just a surrogate of other severe underlying conditions. For example, it was suggested that tricuspid regurgitation could be a sensitive marker of right ventricular dysfunction, or that the presence of tricuspid regurgitation masks the decreased contractility of the right ventricle, analogous to the effect of mitral regurgitation on the ability to estimate left ventricular contractility from left ventricular ejection-fraction [40].

The clinical outcome of patients with functional tricuspid regurgitation secondary to organic mitral valve regurgitation depends to the degree of regurgitation of both valves. The tricuspid regurgitation development can be rapid in the late stages of the mitral disease [41]. This right-side valve regurgitation was initially recognized as a risk factor for early and late mortality after mitral valve surgery [45], even though in later studies right ventricular dysfunction, but not significant tricuspid regurgitation, was independently associated with survival late after left heart valve procedure [18]. Current guidelines support the valve repair for tricuspid regurgitation: both the American College of Cardiology/American Heart Association and the European Society of Cardiology (ESC) guidelines give a class I recommendation for tricuspid valve repair in patients with severe tricuspid regurgitation undergoing mitral valve surgery; ESC guidelines give a class IIa recommendation for concomitant tricuspid valve repair in patients with a tricuspid annular diameter ≥40 mm or moderate tricuspid regurgitation, whereas the American College of Cardiology/American Heart Association gives a more vague, class IIb recommendation for patients with less than severe tricuspid regurgitation [46, 47]. Tricuspid valve annuloplasty is thought to adds little time and complexity to mitral valve surgery and cause only a few further complications [48]; on the contrary, the results of subsequent surgery for isolated late tricuspid regurgitation are poor. Moreover, bioprosthetic valves degenerate with time, and mechanical valves in the tricuspid position cause significant thrombosis events [49]. Some authors reported a 5-fold risk of early death during the perioperative period with tricuspid valve replacement compared with tricuspid valve repair [50]. In some patients with severe organic leaflet involvement, tricuspid valve repair might not be possible, and the valve should be replaced to avoid recurrent severe tricuspid regurgitation or tricuspid stenosis, but with less severe leaflet disease suboptimal results with mild residual tricuspid regurgitation might be well tolerated (in contrast to mitral valve repair, where suboptimal initial results are usually not accepted). Tricuspid valve repair with an annuloplasty ring seems to provide better results as compared to suture annuloplasty [51].

Tricuspid annulus diameter is an essential criterion for ring annuloplasty approach, as the severity of the regurgitation progress with annular diameter increases [52]. Aside from correlation with severity of tricuspid regurgitation, the presence of annular dilation may also be a reflection of a pathologically abnormal valve that is prone to leak in the future and so these dilated annuli may form the substrate for development of late tricuspid regurgitation. The persistence of tricuspid annular dilatation may explain why patients who have had successful mitral valve surgery may still develop severe tricuspid regurgitation several years later despite the absence of pulmonary hypertension. However, it is still uncertain whether annular dilatation is the causative trigger for late tricuspid regurgitation after mitral valve surgery.

Despite the high prevalence, the support of the guidelines, and growing evidence of functional tricuspid regurgitation prognostic importance in patients with left ventricular dysfunction [5, 53], tricuspid valve repair is rarely performed in routine practice for patients with functional tricuspid regurgitation. The correct approach to patients undergoing mitral valve surgery and presenting concomitant tricuspid regurgitation of any degree should include a careful assessment of the tricuspid valve and consideration for potential correction of both the valvular defects.

Functional tricuspid regurgitation may improve after correction of left-sided valvular disease [45], but may also persist or worsen, even in the absence of significant residual mitral regurgitation or other causes of left-sided heart failure [54]. This evolution is still challenging to predict. Tager et al. reported that concomitant tricuspid valve repair at the time of mitral valve surgery results in tricuspid regurgitation resolution in about 85% of patients, and other groups observed a higher incidence of post-operative tricuspid regurgitation in patients in whom tricuspid regurgitation was not treated than in patients who underwent tricuspid valve repair [55]. Furthermore, multiple researchers showed that right ventricular geometry and function improve after tricuspid valve repair at the time of left-sided valve surgery [56, 57]. Unfortunately, the degree of improvement in tricuspid regurgitation after left-sided valvular heart disease correction is still difficult to predict. According to early studies, persistent pulmonary hypertension after mitral valve replacement was implicated as the cause of persisting or worsening tricuspid regurgitation. But this is not the only mechanism, as functional tricuspid regurgitation can persist despite normalization of pulmonary pressures. For example, after successful pulmonary thromboendarterectomy, tricuspid regurgitation persists in up to 30% of patients despite normalization of pulmonary pressure levels [58].

Tricuspid regurgitation could also develop late after mitral valve surgery; this has been reported in up to 40% of patients. Several studies reported a higher long-term mortality rate, lower quality of life, and reduced exercise capacity in patients who develop severe tricuspid regurgitation after mitral valve surgery [59, 60]. On the other hand, survival rate may remain poor despite tricuspid valve surgery, especially in patients presenting with right ventricular systolic dysfunction [61]. Some data suggest that survival rates may be better if surgery is undertaken when patients are in NYHA class II (as opposed to III or IV) and unquestionably before the onset of severe right ventricular dysfunction [62]. For patients undergoing concomitant tricuspid and mitral valve surgery, optimal referral timing is a conundrum and may benefit from a careful assessment of the right ventricular size and function [63]. The potential benefit of other options, such as cardiac transplantation or ventricular assist devices in this patient subgroup, remains undefined.

Considerable uncertainties exist about functional tricuspid regurgitation so that this clinical entity remains highly undertreated in routine practice. In the context of left ventricular dysfunction further studies will need to address whether patients with functional tricuspid regurgitation may benefit from valvular intervention. Similarly, data are needed to refine the correct timing and the appropriate referral criteria for functional tricuspid regurgitation presenting with severe left-valvular disease.

References

[1] Cohen S, Sell J, McIntosh C, Clark R (1987) Tricuspid regurgitation in patients with acquired, chronic, pure mitral regurgitation. II. Nonoperative management, tricuspid valve annuloplasty, and tricuspid valve replacement. *J Thorac Cardiovasc Surg* 94:488–497.

[2] Fox ER, Wilson RS, Penman AD, King JJ, Towery JG, Butler KR, McMullan MR, Skelton TN, Mosley TH, Taylor HA (2007) Epidemiology of pure valvular regurgitation in the large middle-aged African American cohort of the Atherosclerosis Risk in Communities study. *Am Heart J* 154:1229–1234.

[3] d'Arcy JL, Coffey S, Loudon MA, et al. (2016) Large-scale community echocardiographic screening reveals a major burden of undiagnosed valvular heart disease in older people: the OxVALVE Population Cohort Study. *Eur Heart J* 37:3515–3522.

[4] Kazum SS, Sagie A, Shochat T, Ben-Gal T, Bental T, Kornowski R, Shapira Y, Vaturi M, Hasin T (2019) Prevalence, Echocardiographic Correlations, and Clinical Outcome of Tricuspid Regurgitation in Patients with Significant Left Ventricular Dysfunction. *Am J Med* 132:81–87.

[5] Koelling TM, Aaronson KD, Cody RJ, Bach DS, Armstrong WF (2002) Prognostic significance of mitral regurgitation and tricuspid regurgitation in patients with left ventricular systolic dysfunction. *Am Heart J* 144:524–529.

[6] Lancellotti P, Fattouch K, Go YY (2018) Secondary tricuspid regurgitation in patients with left ventricular systolic dysfunction: cause for concern or innocent bystander? *Eur Heart J* 39:3593–3595.

[7] Thenappan T, Gomberg-Maitland M (2014) Epidemiology of pulmonary hypertension and right ventricular failure in left heart failure. *Curr Heart Fail Rep* 11:428–435.

[8] Miller WL, Mahoney DW, Michelena HI, Pislaru SV, Topilsky Y, Enriquez-Sarano M (2011) Contribution of ventricular diastolic dysfunction to pulmonary hypertension complicating chronic systolic heart failure. *JACC Cardiovasc Imaging* 4:946–954.

[9] Szwejkowski BR, Elder DH, Shearer F, Jack D, Choy AMJ, Pringle SD, Struthers AD, George J, Lang CC (2012) Pulmonary hypertension predicts all-cause mortality in patients with heart failure: a retrospective cohort study. *Eur J Heart Fail* 14:162–167.

[10] De Meester P, Van De Bruaene A, Herijgers P, Voigt JU, Budts W (2012) Tricuspid valve regurgitation: prevalence and relationship with different types of heart disease. *Acta Cardiol* 67:549–556.

[11] Koukoui D, Monakier D, Vaturi M, Shpira Y, Weisenberg D, Yosef D, Sagie A (2008) Natural history and clinical significance of tricuspid regurgitation in patients with mitral valve prolapse and significant mitral regurgitation. *55th Annu. Conf. Isr. Heart Soc. Tel* Aviv Isr.

[12] Matsunaga A, Duran CMG (2005) Progression of tricuspid regurgitation after repaired functional ischemic mitral regurgitation. *Circulation* 112:I453-457.

[13] Waller BF, Morrow AG, Maron BJ, Del Negro AA, Kent KM, McGrath FJ, Wallace RB, McIntosh CL, Roberts WC (1982) Etiology of clinically isolated, severe, chronic, pure mitral regurgitation: analysis of 97 patients over 30 years of age having mitral valve replacement. *Am Heart J* 104:276–288.

[14] Yilmaz O, Suri RM, Dearani JA, Sundt III TM, Daly RC, Burkhart HM, Li Z, Enriquez-Sarano M, Schaff HV (2011) Functional tricuspid regurgitation at the time of mitral valve repair for degenerative leaflet prolapse: the case for a selective approach. *J Thorac Cardiovasc Surg* 142:608–613.

[15] Dreyfus GD, Corbi PJ, Chan KMJ, Bahrami T (2005) Secondary tricuspid regurgitation or dilatation: which should be the criteria for surgical repair? *Ann Thorac Surg* 79:127–132.

[16] Scampardonis G, YANG SS, Maranhão V, Goldberg H, Gooch AS (1973) Left ventricular abnormalities in prolapsed mitral leaflet syndrome: Review of eighty-seven cases. *Circulation* 48:287–297.

[17] Weyman AE, Scherrer-Crosbie M (2004) Marfan syndrome and mitral valve prolapse. *J Clin Invest* 114:1543–1546.

[18] Kammerlander AA, Marzluf BA, Graf A, Bachmann A, Kocher A, Bonderman D, Mascherbauer J (2014) Right ventricular dysfunction, but not tricuspid regurgitation, is associated with outcome late after left heart valve procedure. *J Am Coll Cardiol* 64:2633–2642.

[19] Dreyfus GD, Martin RP, Chan KJ, Dulguerov F, Alexandrescu C (2015) Functional tricuspid regurgitation: a need to revise our understanding. *J Am Coll Cardiol* 65:2331–2336.

[20] Nagel E, Stuber M, Hess O (1996) Importance of the right ventricle in valvular heart disease. *Eur Heart J* 17:829–836.

[21] Antunes MJ, Rodríguez-Palomares J, Prendergast B, et al. (2017) Management of tricuspid valve regurgitation: Position statement of the European Society of Cardiology Working Groups of Cardiovascular Surgery and Valvular Heart Disease. *Eur J Cardiothorac Surg* 52:1022–1030.

[22] Badano LP, Muraru D, Enriquez-Sarano M (2013) Assessment of functional tricuspid regurgitation. *Eur Heart J* 34:1875–1885.

[23] Fukuda S, Gillinov AM, Song JM, Daimon M, Kongsaerepong V, Thomas JD, Shiota T (2006) Echocardiographic insights into atrial and ventricular mechanisms of functional tricuspid regurgitation. *Am Heart J* 152:1208–1214.

[24] Utsunomiya H, Itabashi Y, Mihara H, Berdejo J, Kobayashi S, Siegel RJ, Shiota T (2017) Functional tricuspid regurgitation caused by chronic atrial fibrillation: a real-time 3-dimensional transesophageal echocardiography study. *Circ Cardiovasc Imaging* 10:e004897.

[25] Sallach JA, Tang WW, Borowski AG, Tong W, Porter T, Martin MG, Jasper SE, Shrestha K, Troughton RW, Klein AL (2009) Right atrial volume index in chronic systolic heart failure and prognosis. *JACC Cardiovasc Imaging* 2:527–534.

[26] Miller WL, Grill DE, Borlaug BA (2013) Clinical features, hemodynamics, and outcomes of pulmonary hypertension due to chronic heart failure with reduced ejection fraction: pulmonary hypertension and heart failure. *JACC Heart Fail* 1:290–299.

[27] Tribouilloy C, Enriquez-Sarano M, Rossi A, Tajik A, Seward J (1997) Determinants of the pulmonary artery pressure rise in left ventricular dysfunction. *Cardiol Rome Italy* 42:1051–1058.

[28] Mutlak D, Aronson D, Lessick J, Reisner SA, Dabbah S, Agmon Y (2009) Functional tricuspid regurgitation in patients with pulmonary hypertension: Is pulmonary artery pressure the only determinant of regurgitation severity? *Chest* 135:115–121.

[29] Rogers JH, Bolling SF (2009) The tricuspid valve: Current perspective and evolving management of tricuspid regurgitation. *Circulation* 119:2718–2725.

[30] Katsi V, Raftopoulos L, Aggeli C, Vlasseros I, Felekos I, Tousoulis D, Stefanadis C, Kallikazaros I (2012) Tricuspid regurgitation after successful mitral valve surgery. *Interact Cardiovasc Thorac Surg* 15:102–108.

[31] Goldstone AB, Howard JL, Cohen JE, MacArthur Jr JW, Atluri P, Kirkpatrick JN, Woo YJ (2014) Natural history of coexistent tricuspid regurgitation in patients with degenerative mitral valve

disease: implications for future guidelines. *J Thorac Cardiovasc Surg* 148:2802–2810.

[32] Roberts WC, Eways EA (1991) Clinical and anatomic observations in patients having mitral valve replacement for pure mitral regurgitation and simultaneous tricuspid valve replacement. *Am J Cardiol* 68:1107–1111.

[33] Ubago JL, Figueroa A, Ochoteco A, Colman T, Duran RM, Duran CG (1983) Analysis of the amount of tricuspid valve anular dilatation required to produce functional tricuspid regurgitation. *Am J Cardiol* 52:155–158.

[34] Kocica MJ, Corno AF, Carreras-Costa F, Ballester-Rodes M, Moghbel MC, Cueva CN, Lackovic V, Kanjuh VI, Torrent-Guasp F (2006) The helical ventricular myocardial band: global, three-dimensional, functional architecture of the ventricular myocardium. *Eur J Cardiothorac Surg* 29:S21–S40.

[35] Sallin EA (1969) Fiber orientation and ejection fraction in the human left ventricle. *Biophys J* 9:954–964.

[36] Suga H, Sagawa K, Shoukas AA (1973) Load independence of the instantaneous pressure-volume ratio of the canine left ventricle and effects of epinephrine and heart rate on the ratio. *Circ Res* 32:314–322.

[37] Buckberg G, Hoffman JI (2014) Right ventricular architecture responsible for mechanical performance: unifying role of ventricular septum. *J Thorac Cardiovasc Surg* 148:3166–3171.

[38] Bueno H, López-Palop R, Bermejo J, López-Sendón JL, Delcán JL (1997) In-hospital outcome of elderly patients with acute inferior myocardial infarction and right ventricular involvement. *Circulation* 96:436–441.

[39] Flett AS, Sado DM, Quarta G, et al. (2012) Diffuse myocardial fibrosis in severe aortic stenosis: an equilibrium contrast cardiovascular magnetic resonance study. *Eur Heart Journal–Cardiovascular Imaging* 13:819–826.

[40] Nath J, Foster E, Heidenreich PA (2004) Impact of Tricuspid Regurgitation on Long-Term Survival. *J Am Coll Cardiol* 43:405–409.

[41] Vahanian A PJ Pierard L, Dion R (2009) Valvular heart disease. In: *ESC Textb. Cardiovasc. Med.* Oxford University Press, pp 763–817.

[42] D'alonzo GE, Barst RJ, Ayres SM, et al. (1991) Survival in patients with primary pulmonary hypertension: results from a national prospective registry. *Ann Intern Med* 115:343–349.

[43] Weitsman T, Weisz G, Farkash R, Klutstein M, Butnaru A, Rosenmann D, Hasin T (2017) Pulmonary hypertension with left heart disease: prevalence, temporal shifts in etiologies and outcome. *Am J Med* 130:1272–1279.

[44] Topilsky Y, Khanna A, Le Toumeau T, Park S, Michelena H, Suri R, Mahoney DW, Enriquez-Sarano M (2012) Clinical context and mechanism of functional tricuspid regurgitation in patients with and without pulmonary hypertension. *Circ Cardiovasc Imaging* 5:314–323.

[45] Braunwald NS, Ross JR J, Morrow AG (1967) Conservative management of tricuspid regurgitation in patients undergoing mitral valve replacement. *Circulation* 35:I–63.

[46] Baumgartner H, Falk V, Bax JJ, et al. (2017) 2017 ESC/EACTS guidelines for the management of valvular heart disease. *Eur Heart J* 38:2739–2791.

[47] Nishimura RA, Otto C (2014) *2014 ACC/AHA valve guidelines: earlier intervention for chronic mitral regurgitation*. BMJ Publishing Group Ltd and British Cardiovascular Society.

[48] Singh G, Singh SK, König A, Reutlinger K, Nye MD, Adhikary T, Eilers M, Gress TM, Fernandez-Zapico ME, Ellenrieder V (2010) Sequential activation of NFAT and c-Myc transcription factors mediates the TGF-beta switch from a suppressor to a promoter of cancer cell proliferation. *J Biol Chem* 285:27241–27250.

[49] Chang B-C, Lim S-H, Yi G, Hong YS, Lee S, Yoo K-J, Kang MS, Cho BK (2006) Long-term clinical results of tricuspid valve replacement. *Ann Thorac Surg* 81:1317–1324.

[50] Antunes MJ, Barlow JB (2007) Management of tricuspid valve regurgitation. *Heart* 93:271–276.

[51] Singh SK, Tang GH, Maganti MD, Armstrong S, Williams WG, David TE, Borger MA (2006) Midterm outcomes of tricuspid valve repair versus replacement for organic tricuspid disease. *Ann Thorac Surg* 82:1735–1741.

[52] Sugimoto T, Okada M, Ozaki N, Hatakeyama T, Kawahira T (1999) Long-term evaluation of treatment for functional tricuspid regurgitation with regurgitant volume: characteristic differences based on primary cardiac lesion. *J Thorac Cardiovasc Surg* 117:463–471.

[53] Hung J, Koelling T, Semigran MJ, Dec GW, Levine RA, Di Salvo TG (1998) Usefulness of echocardiographic determined tricuspid regurgitation in predicting event-free survival in severe heart failure secondary to idiopathic-dilated cardiomyopathy or to ischemic cardiomyopathy. *Am J Cardiol* 82:1301–1303.

[54] King RM, Schaff HV, Danielson GK, Gersh BJ, Orszulak TA, Piehler JM, Puga FJ, Pluth JR (1984) Surgery for tricuspid regurgitation late after mitral valve replacement. *Circulation* 70:I193–7.

[55] Tager R, Skudicky D, Mueller U, Essop R, Hammond G, Sareli P (1998) Long-term follow-up of rheumatic patients undergoing left-sided valve replacement with tricuspid annuloplasty—validity of preoperative echocardiographic criteria in the decision to perform tricuspid annuloplasty. *Am J Cardiol* 81:1013–1016.

[56] Desai AR, Branco RG, Comitis GA, Maiya S, Vyas DB, Vaz Silva P, Sethia B, Slavik Z, Larovere JM (2013) Early Postoperative Outcomes Following Surgical Repair of Complete Atrioventricular Septal Defects: Is Down Syndrome a Risk Factor? *Pediatr Crit Care Med J Soc Crit Care Med World Fed Pediatr Intensive Crit Care Soc.* doi: 10.1097/PCC.0000000000000004.

[57] Bertrand PB, Koppers G, Verbrugge FH, Mullens W, Vandervoort P, Dion R, Verhaert D (2014) Tricuspid annuloplasty concomitant with

mitral valve surgery: effects on right ventricular remodeling. *J Thorac Cardiovasc Surg* 147:1256–1264.

[58] Menzel T, Kramm T, Wagner S, Mohr-Kahaly S, Mayer E, Meyer J (2002) Improvement of tricuspid regurgitation after pulmonary thromboendarterectomy. *Ann Thorac Surg* 73:756–761.

[59] Sagie A, Schwammenthal E, Palacios IF, King ME, Leavitt M, Freitas N, Weyman AE, Levine RA (1994) Significant tricuspid regurgitation does not resolve after percutaneous balloon mitral valvotomy. *J Thorac Cardiovasc Surg* 108:727–735.

[60] Matsuyama K, Matsumoto M, Sugita T, Nishizawa J, Tokuda Y, Matsuo T (2003) Predictors of residual tricuspid regurgitation after mitral valve surgery. *Ann Thorac Surg* 75:1826–1828.

[61] Kim YJ, Kwon DA, Kim HK, et al. (2009) Determinants of surgical outcome in patients with isolated tricuspid regurgitation. *Circulation* 120(17):1672-8.

[62] Kwon DA, Park JS, Chang HJ, Kim YJ, Sohn DW, Kim KB, Ahn H, Oh BH, Park YB, Choi YS (2006) Prediction of outcome in patients undergoing surgery for severe tricuspid regurgitation following mitral valve surgery and role of tricuspid annular systolic velocity. *Am J Cardiol* 98:659–661.

[63] Yiu KH, Wong A, Pu L, et al. (2014) Prognostic value of preoperative right ventricular geometry and tricuspid valve tethering area in patients undergoing tricuspid annuloplasty. *Circulation* 129:87–92.

In: The Rediscovered Tricuspid Valve ISBN: 978-1-53616-098-7
Editor: Giacomo Bianchi

Chapter 7

TRICUSPID VALVE ENDOCARDITIS: EPIDEMIOLOGY, TREATMENT AND OUTCOMES

Enrico Tagliaferri**, *MD
Department of Infectious Disease, University of Pisa, Pisa, Italy

ABSTRACT

Right-sided endocarditis, although accounting for only 5-10% of all cases of infective endocarditis, bear major risk of mortality and morbidity as well as chronic sequelae. Although *Staphylococcus aureus* is responsible for a significant proportion of cases, although complex pathogen-host interaction and setting-specific enviromental factors sustain the infection from other procariotes and also yeasts and molds. The approach to the patient with right-sided endocarditis involves the integration of clinical suspicion and probability of endocarditis, supported by the use of blood tests and imaging. Antibiotic treatment is a fundamental cornerstone in the patient's therapeutic pathway, although in some cases surgical remediation cannot be avoided to eradicate the infection or to treat local and systemic complications.

* Corresponding Author's E-mail: e.tagliaferri@ao-pisa.toscana.it.

Keywords: native valve; tricuspid valve; endocarditis, virulence; outcome

INTRODUCTION

Right-sided infective endocarditis (RSIE) accounts for 5–10% of all cases of infective endocarditis (IE) [1, 2]. The majority of cases involves the tricuspid valve. Well known risk factors are intravenous drug abuse and intravascular devices, particularly central venous catheters and cardiovascular implantable electronic devices (CIED) [3, 4].

The fact that RSIE has a much lower incidence than left-sided infective endocarditis (LSIE) [1, 5] could be due to:

(a) low incidence of congenital disease on the right side of the heart; in a retrospective study [6] of 16 patients with endocarditis and congenital heart defects only six had tricuspid valve disease;
(b) low hemodynamic pressure on the tricuspid and pulmonary valves;
(c) low oxygen saturation.

The management of RSIE among intravenous drug users (IDUs) poses a significant challenge, particularly when combined with human immunodeficiency virus (HIV) or hepatitis C virus infection, due to high burden of co-morbidity and concomitant medications. Although RSIE prognosis is generally more favorable than that of LSIE, 5–16% of cases will eventually require surgery [7–9]. There is no definite general consensus on the best surgical approach, that is also influenced by poor postoperative compliance and high relapse rate among IDUs.

EPIDEMIOLOGY

Most cases of RSIE involve the tricuspid valve, while isolated pulmonary valve involvement is rare [10]. Isolated cases of RSIE involving the eustachian valve, interventricular septum or right ventricular free wall have also been reported [1, 11].

Intravenous drug abuse is the main risk factor and it's responsible for the increasing incidence in high-income countries, while in low-income countries, septic abortion and intra-abdominal sepsis are still important risk factors [1, 12, 13]. Up to 86% of IE cases among IDUs are RSIE cases and around 90% of them involve the tricuspid valve [11].

RSIE in non-IDU accounts for only 9% of all cases of IE. Intravascular catheters, CIEDs and other intracardiac devices, such as catheters for hemodialysis or tricuspid prosthetic valve, are the commonest predisposing factors [3, 8, 13–15]. Nonetheless, even among patients with intracardiac hemodialysis catheters entering the right atrium or distal arteriovenous shunts, tricuspid valve endocarditis occurs in a minority of cases; according to data from the Society of Thoracic Surgery, between January 1994 and December 2003, including a total of 1,862 valvular procedures in dialysis patients with endocarditis, isolated tricuspid valve was recorded in 55 cases (3%) [16, 17].

MICROBIOLOGY

Staphylococcus aureus is the major microbiological cause of RSIE in both IDUs and non-addicts [2, 14].

Other causes of RSIE include coagulase-negative staphylococci and streptococci [14]. *Lactobacillus spp.*, HACEK organisms (*Haemophilus aphrophilus, Actinobacillus actinomycetemcomitans, Cardiobacterium hominis, Eikenella corrodens* and *Kingella kingae*), *Enterococcus spp.*

Yeasts and molds have also been reported as infrequent causes of RSIE [1, 2, 11, 18]. Fungi are responsible for relatively few (3%) of all cases of IE, but only rarely (7%) located to the right side of the heart [19]. IDU as a risk factor for fungal IE is only described in a minority (4–13%) of cases, caused by *Candida spp.* or in a few cases by *Aspergillus spp.*, occasionally seen in the presence of HIV [20].

Unfortunately, in the setting of healthcare-associated infections, such as those affecting patients with indwelling devices, Gram negative bacilli (GNB) can be responsible of RSIE in the course of bacteremia, especially if infection is not timely diagnosed and managed and devices are not promptly removed. In this setting, a particularly serious challenge is represented by multidrug-resistant (MDR) microorganisms such as *Acinetobacter baumannii*, *Pseudomonas aeruginosa* and *Enterobacteriaceae* producing extended spectrum beta-lactamase (ESBL) and carbapenemase. In a contemporary multicenter cohort of 58 patients with IE due to GNB, prospectively observed in 26 Italian centers from 2004 to 2011, *Escherichia coli* was the most common pathogen, followed by *Pseudomonas aeruginosa* and *Klebsiella pneumoniae*. The genitourinary tract as a source of infection, immunosuppression, and the presence of a CIED were independently associated with IE due to GNB. In-hospital mortality was 13.8%, and mortality rose to 30.6% at 1 year. A MDR etiology was associated with in-hospital mortality and 1-year mortality [21].

Cases of IE, including RSIE, due to KPC-carbapenemase producing *K. pneumoniae* have been described [22, 23].

Clinical Manifestations and Diagnosis

The diagnosis of RSIE should always be considered in IDUs and patients with indwelling devices presenting with symptoms and signs of infection.

Clinical presentation usually includes respiratory symptoms and fever, chills, weight loss and weakness [24]. Compared to LSIE, diagnosis of RSIE is often delayed, since right-sided murmurs often go undetected and peripheral signs of embolism are absent. In contrast to LSIE, pulmonary embolism occurs in 75–100%, especially in case of tricuspid valve IE [5]. Differential diagnosis includes pulmonary embolism, pulmonary tumor and interstitial or lobar pneumonia of any cause, including aspiration pneumonia and hypersensitivity pneumonitis [5, 25].

Blood Tests and Specific Cultures

Blood cultures, according to modified Duke's criteria, are the cornerstone for diagnosis. Therefore, antimicrobial therapy for suspected RSIE should be initiated after adequate blood cultures have been obtained. At least three sets of blood cultures (one bottle for aerobes and one for anaerobes) should be taken inoculating 10 ml of blood in each bottle. If the patient is clinically stable, waiting 24-48 hours before starting antibiotic treatment, to take more samples in a wider span of time should be considered. Infection due to fastidious pathogens or prior administration of antibiotics can result in negative blood cultures [26].

Remarkably, blood culture sensibility in invasive candidiasis stands around 50% in various studies [27]. To overcome this obstacle, nonculture-based diagnostic tests have been developed for detection in blood of components of the fungal cell wall (such as mannan and β-d-glucan (BDG)) by immunoassays, of DNA by polymerase chain reaction (PCR), and of antibodies by serology. The performance of BDG assays in invasive fungal infections has been assessed in three systematic reviews. In the subgroup of patients with proven infection, the pooled sensitivities and specificities of BDG were 79.1%, 87.7%, and 78%, respectively [28–30]. Importantly, BDG assays are not species-specific so further tests are needed to identify the fungus. In patients with suspected invasive candidiasis, the presence of elevated circulating levels of *Candida* mannan antigen in the blood had a sensitivity of 58% and a specificity of 93% [31]. In the same group of patients, the detection of anti-mannan antibodies had a sensitivity of 59% and a specificity of 83%. The sensitivity increased to 83% when the mannan and anti-mannan assays were combined, but the specificity remained similar at 86%. PCRs for fungi continue to be challenging for technical reasons and there are no commercially available tests at present. However, in a review of more than 50 standard, nested, or real-time PCRs [32], the pooled sensitivity and specificity were 95% and 92%, respectively, for invasive candidiasis and the current trends in microbiology suggest a probable major contribution of test based on nucleic acid detection, also in this setting.

Routine blood tests are non-specific but white blood cells (WBC) count, erythrosedimentation rate (ESR) and C-reactive protein (CRP) are usually increased; leucopoenia can be detected instead in cases of sepsis; anemia and microscopic hematuria can often be demonstrated [24]. In case of sepsis, laboratory signs of organ failure can be present.

Instrumental Diagnostic Tests

Electrocardiography

In this setting, the use of surface electrocardiogram (EKG) is non-specific and does not rise suspicion unless extensive involvement of the subvalvular apparatus and conduction system are involved.

Chest X-Ray and Computed Tomography

Chest X-ray can reveal findings of pulmonary embolism due to septic emboli from the right heart [11]. Chest computed tomography scan (CT-scan) can demonstrate multiple infiltrates with cavities in both lungs, suggesting the presence of multiple pulmonary embolisms and lung abscesses [5, 8].

Multislice computed tomography (MSCT) can be used to detect abscesses/pseudoaneurysms with a diagnostic accuracy similar to TEE, and is possibly superior in the provision of information regarding the extent and consequences of any perivalvular extension, including the anatomy of pseudoaneurysms, abscesses and fistulae [33].

Ultrasounds

Transesophageal echocardiography (TEE) has been reported by some not to improve diagnostic accuracy of transthoracic echocardiography (TTE), as in LSIE, in the detection of vegetations associated with RSIE in IDUs [34]. However, TEE may prove more sensitive in detecting vegetations on pulmonary valves, central intravenous catheters and CIEDs, prosthetic valve endocarditis, foreign bodies, unusual locations of RSIE and complications such as perivalvular abscesses [24]. The diagnosis of

CIED endocarditis is based on the finding of lead and/or valvular vegetations through the TEE and has been identified in 18–23% of the cases [4, 8, 35]. Updated guidelines recommend TEE to be performed in all cases of suspected endocarditis and negative or non-diagnostic TTE [36]. In all patients with *S. aureus* bacteremia, echocardiography is justified in view of the frequency of IE in this setting, the virulence of this organism and its devastating effects once intracardiac infection is established [37, 38].

Real-time three-dimensional (3D) TEE allows the analysis of 3D volumes of cardiac structures in any possible plane. A recent study has shown that conventional TEE underestimates vegetation size and that 3D TEE is a feasible technique for the analysis of vegetation morphology and size that may overcome the shortcomings of conventional TEE, leading to a better prediction of the embolic risk in IE [39].

In recent years, a possible role of Intracardiac Echocardiography (ICE) has been proposed. In the study of Narducci et al. 152 patients with CIED infection underwent transvenous lead extraction; using the modified Duke criteria, they were divided into 3 groups: 44 with a "definite" diagnosis of IE (group 1), 52 with a "possible" diagnosis of IE (group 2), and 56 with a "rejected" diagnosis of IE (group 3); ICE shows high diagnostic accuracy in the detection of intracardiac masses (ICM) among patients with a definite diagnosis of cardiac device–related IE, while in patients with a clinical suspicion of device-related IE undergoing transvenous lead extraction, ICE provided a significantly higher diagnostic power for the detection of ICM compared with TEE; according to the authors ICE represents a useful technique for the diagnosis of ICM, thus providing improved imaging of right-sided leads and increasing the diagnostic yield compared with TEE [40].

Radionuclide Studies

The ventilation/perfusion scan of the lungs may be useful in detecting septic pulmonary emboli in some cases [8].

Radiolabeled white blood cell (WBC) SPECT/CT and ^{18}F-FDG PET/CT have been described to play a significant role in the diagnosis of

IE. These techniques are able to detect possible infective foci at cardiac level and at the same time peripheral embolic and metastatic infectious events [41]. Caution must be exercised when interpreting ^{18}F-FDG PET/CT results in patients who have recently undergone cardiac surgery, as a postoperative inflammatory response may result in non-specific ^{18}F-FDG uptake in the immediate postoperative period. A number of pathological conditions can mimic the pattern of focally increased ^{18}F-FDG uptake, such as active thrombi, soft atherosclerotic plaques, vasculitis, primary cardiac tumors, cardiac metastasis from a non-cardiac tumor, post-surgical inflammation and foreign body reactions [42]. Radiolabeled WBC SPECT/CT is more specific for the detection of IE and infectious foci than ^{18}F-FDG PET/CT and should be preferred in all situations that require enhanced specificity [43]. Disadvantages of scintigraphy with radiolabeled WBC are the requirement of blood handling, the duration of the procedure, which is more time consuming than PET/CT, and a slightly lower spatial resolution and photon detection efficiency compared with PET/CT. An additional role of ^{18}F-FDG PET/CT may be seen in the follow up of patients with IE to monitor response to antimicrobial treatment.

In facts, abnormal activity around the site of prosthetic valve implantation detected by ^{18}F-FDG PET/CT (if the prosthesis was implanted at least 3 months before) or radiolabeled leukocytes SPECT/CT and definite paravalvular lesions by cardiac CT are now considered major criteria for the diagnosis of endocarditis by the European Society of Cardiology (Table 1) [36].

As a reminder, *definite IE* is diagnosed in presence of pathological criteria (microorganisms demonstrated by culture or on histological examination of a vegetation, a vegetation that has embolized, or an intracardiac abscess specimen; or pathological lesions such as vegetation or intracardiac abscess confirmed by histological examination showing active endocarditis) or clinical criteria (2 major criteria; or 1 major criterion and 3 minor criteria; or 5 minor criteria). *Possible IE* is defined by 1 major criterion and 1 minor criterion; or 3 minor criteria. Diagnosis of IE is rejected in case of firm alternate diagnosis; or resolution of symptoms suggesting IE with antibiotic therapy for $\leq$4 days; or no pathological evidence of IE at surgery or autopsy, with antibiotic therapy for ≤4 days; or does not meet criteria for possible IE, as above [36].

Table 1. Modified duke criteria for the diagnosis of infective endocarditis

Major Criteria	Minor Criteria
Blood cultures positive for IE a. Typical microorganisms consistent with IE from 2 separate blood cultures b. Microorganisms consistent with IE from persistently positive blood cultures c. Single positive blood culture for *C. burnetiid* or phase I IgG antibody titer >1:800 Imaging positive for IE 1. Echocardiogram positive for IE 2. Abnormal activity around the site of prosthetic valve implantation detected by ^{18}F-FDG PET/CT or radiolabeled WBC 3. Definite paravalvular lesions by cardiac CT	1. Predisposition such as predisposing heart condition, or injection drug use 2. Fever defined as temperature >38°C 3. Vascular phenomena 4. Immunological phenomena 5. Microbiological evidence

ANTIBIOTIC TREATMENT

Empirical therapy should be targeted at the most likely causative organisms and therefore include anti-staphylococcal agents with activity against methicillin resistant *S. aureus* (MRSA) such as the combination of vancomycin and gentamicin, or daptomycin alone. Once culture and sensitivity results of an identified microorganism are known, antibiotic therapy can be appropriately modified, lasting up to 6 weeks [18].

In case methicillin-susceptible *S. aureus* (MSSA) is isolated, oxacillin or cefazolin are the drugs of choice, since they are bactericidal and well tolerated. Notably, in a large, multicenter study, patients who received cefazolin had a lower risk of mortality and similar odds of recurrent infections compared with nafcillin or oxacillin for MSSA infections complicated by bacteremia [44].

In case of staphylococcal endocarditis on a prosthetic valve, betalactam or anti-MRSA agent, according to the underlying pathogen, should be combined with rifampin and gentamicin (the latter for two weeks) [36]. Also, gentamicin can be given in a single daily dose in order to maximize its concentration-dependent activity and to reduce renal toxicity [45]. Starting rifampin 3–5 days later than vancomycin and gentamicin has been suggested by some experts in order to protect rifampin by selection of resistance [46].

In endocarditis, as paradigm of a hard-to-treat infection, therapeutic drug monitoring (TDM) is crucial to ensure adequate blood levels of antibiotics are obtained, in order to optimize bactericidal activity and minimize risk of side effects; TDM is widely available for daptomycin, gentamicin and vancomycin [8, 12, 14, 15].

Treatment of streptococcal endocarditis usually relies on a combination of a beta-lactam, such as penicillin, amoxicillin or ceftriaxone, with gentamicin. While traditional therapy of endocarditis due to *Enterococcus faecalis* is based on ampicillin plus gentamicin, in recent years, the combination of ampicillin and ceftriaxone has been demonstrated to be synergistic *in vitro*, effective *in vivo* and better tolerated than ampicillin plus gentamicin [47].

In the management of infections due to MDR micro-organisms combination treatment is generally adopted, sometimes including off-label regimes; infections due to KPC-producing *K. pneumoniae* are usually managed with various combinations including colistin, fosfomycin, aminoglycosides and high-dose tigecycline. Recently, the availability of compounds active against MDR Gram negative bacteria, such as ceftazidime/avibactam for KPC-producing *K. pneumoniae* and ceftolozane/tazobactam for ESBL-producing *Enterobacteriaceae* and MDR *P. aeruginosa*, has improved significantly the management of these cases. Infectious Diseases consultant should systematically be involved. While some combinations of antibiotics have a known synergistic effect, others may have variable interactions that should be first assessed in vitro.

Synergy testing can be performed with various methods, including time-kill curves, checkerboard, and methods using Kirby Bauer diskettes, Etest strips and antibiotic-added solid media plates [48].

In the setting of endocarditis, the assessment of bactericidal activity of the therapy regimen is necessary. Bacteriostatic and bactericidal activity of serum of patients on treatment can be titred against the bug isolated from blood cultures. Additionally, activity of the serum can be tested before and after adding an agent to the combination to confirm a possible advantage [49].

Treatment of Candida endocarditis can be particularly challenging. Lipid formulation Amphotericin B, 3–5 mg/kg daily, with or without flucytosine, 25 mg/kg 4 times daily, or high-dose echinocandin (caspofungin 150 mg daily, micafungin 150 mg daily, or anidulafungin 200 mg daily) is recommended as initial therapy. Step-down therapy to fluconazole, 400–800 mg (6–12 mg/kg) daily, may be considered for patients who have susceptible isolates, are clinically stable, and have cleared Candida from the bloodstream. Valve replacement is recommended; treatment should continue for at least 6 weeks after surgery and for a longer duration in patients with perivalvular abscesses and other complications. For patients who cannot undergo valve replacement, long-term suppression with fluconazole is recommended [50].

The duration of antibiotic treatment after surgery is not definitely established. Four to six weeks of the pre-operatively selected antibiotic, irrespective of etiologic factors, has been suggested. Nevertheless, shorter duration of postoperative treatment does not necessarily lead to a higher incidence of relapse, if certain criteria are fulfilled (i.e., negative valve cultures, adequate compliance) making a 2-week scheme of postoperative treatment probably adequate. Probably, the maximum period of postoperative antibiotic administration (4–6 weeks) should be considered in cases of: (a) annular involvement, (b) implantation of prosthetic material (ring or non-homograft valve), (c) postoperative presence of significant regurgitation, (d) IDUs, (e) non-radical debridement, (f) extracardiac sites of infection, (g) positive culture of extracted material or valve and (h) etiology of staphylococci, GNB and fungi. In non-IDUs with none of the above criteria, 2 weeks of post-operative antibiotic therapy should be sufficient [51].

Indications for Surgical Treatment, Timing of Intervention and Outcomes

Early surgical experience led to the idea that RSIE can be managed with medical treatment alone in 70–85% of cases [52, 53].

Though there is no definitive consensus, indications can be summarized as follows : (a) persistent signs of infection after two weeks of antibiotic therapy, except for pathogens for which aggressive treatment should be considered earlier (*S. aureus*, Gram negative rods and fungi); (b) recurrent septic pulmonary embolism; (c) massive or worsening tricuspid regurgitation contributing to deteriorating heart failure; (d) septic shock (indication for emergency surgery); (e) when the size of a vegetation increases or persists in spite of appropriate antibiotic treatment at >1 cm; (f) new-onset or worsening renal or hepatic failure; (g) multivalvular involvement; and (h) following failure or complications of percutaneous removal of infected CIED [12, 53–55]. About this, although some studies do not support percutaneous lead extraction when vegetation size extends >10 mm [3, 15], Mayo Clinic advocates successful and safe percutaneous removal of device components in nearly all patients [8].

Timing of surgical management depends on the following factors: (a) cause of endocarditis (urgent in CIED endocarditis or prosthetic tricuspid endocarditis), (b) etiology (fungal, Gram negative rods, MRSA, etc.), (c) coexistence with LSIE, (e) response to antibiotic treatment, (f) toxicity of antibiotics and (g) complications (abscess, increased vegetation's size, etc.) [3, 4, 8, 34, 35, 52, 55, 56]. Early surgery should be considered if *S. aureus* is suspected. *S. aureus* infections are often complicated infections with large vegetations, aggressive valve destruction and embolic manifestations resulting in an increased risk of mortality [52]. Medical management alone of staphylococcal endocarditis was associated with higher mortality (51%)

than combined medical/surgical therapy (31%) [57]. Particularly, if multi-resistant *S. aureus* is detected, surgery is often the only conclusive therapy [58].

A fungal cause often goes undiagnosed for a long time due to persistently negative blood cultures. Overall survival of fungal endocarditis with antifungals alone barely reaches 25%, whereas a combination of medical/surgical management can increase it up to 58% [59].

Several other uncommon microorganisms such as *Brucella spp*, *Coxiella burnetii* and *Pseudomonas aeruginosa* indicate surgical intervention, especially due to the associated comorbidities [61-63] [60–62]. In the absence of LSIE, early surgery should be considered in the presence of life-threatening complications such as severe congestive heart failure, abscess or massive pulmonary emboli. Large tricuspid valve vegetations (>2 cm), especially in the context of mycotic endocarditis, are related to valve insufficiency and pulmonary embolization that predict a poor outcome [10, 63].

Persistent sepsis despite antibiotic treatment demands surgical intervention [64]. However, a persistent fever associated with respiratory symptoms may continue for weeks despite appropriate antibiotic management, but does ultimately respond [10, 65]. Therefore, blood cultures play a key role also in the follow-up to identify patients who are persistently bacteremic, demonstrating that therapy is not effective.

The general objectives of surgery in the setting of RSIE are: (a) radical debridement of vegetations and infected tissue, (b) avoidance of implantation of prosthetic material, especially in IDU, and (c) correction of valve regurgitation [7, 57, 66–68].

Surgical techniques can be divided into those that utilize prosthetic material for repair or replacement and those that use native or autologous material.

In IDUs who have a high risk of complications due to low compliance with anticoagulant therapy and reinfection related to resumption of drug abuse [69, 70], vegetectomy and valve repair avoiding artificial material should be considered the first line of surgical management [7]. If this is not technically feasible, then tricuspid valve replacement should be performed [71].

OUTCOMES

The reported surgical mortality rate for patients with infective endocarditis has improved from 30% in the 1970s to 7.4–9.9% in the 2000s [72].

The 20-year survival rate after RSIE operation was 58%, falling to 36% for patients with left as well as right-sided involvement [7]. Similarly, surgical mortality in IDUs with RSIE is less than 2% [73]. Reoperation rates for recurrent endocarditis seem to be significantly higher in IDUs (17%) versus non-IDUs (5%) [74]. Survival rates at 10- and 15-years following valve replacement levels were 66 and 54% for IDUs and 56 and 42% for non-IDUs, probably due to the younger age group of IDU [74]. Comparison of valve repair and replacement remains challenging, also because valve repair is recommended in milder cases. In a study of 22 patients with tricuspid endocarditis, surgical mortality as well as complication rates (relapse, reoperation) were higher in the replacement group, confirming that valve replacement should be considered only when repair is considered inappropriate [54, 75]. Long-term results of replacement (106 patients) and repair (310 patients) in a total of 416 patients with tricuspid valve pathology showed that: (a) surgical mortality in the repair and the replacement group were 13.9 versus 33%, (b) replacement was an independent risk factor for operative mortality, (c) 10-year actuarial survival was significantly higher in the repair group (47 versus 37.4%) and (d) the incidence of reoperation was equally low. Following these results, these authors recommend the use of a biological prosthesis following tricuspid valve replacement [76]. Singh et al. compared midterm results following repair (178 patients) or replacement (78 patients) of tricuspid valve due to organic disease; tricuspid valve repair was associated with better perioperative, midterm and event-free survival than tricuspid valve replacement in patients with organic tricuspid disease. Despite more tricuspid regurgitation in the repair group during follow-up, reoperation rates and functional class were similar [77]. These results disagree with a meta-analysis performed by Moraca et al. comparing a matched cohort of patients undergoing repair versus replacement using propensity score analysis (68 patients in each group): no significant difference in surgical mortality and 10-year survival was observed, so that the authors recommend tricuspid valve replacement for patients in whom there is a reasonable chance for recurrence of regurgitation after repair [78].

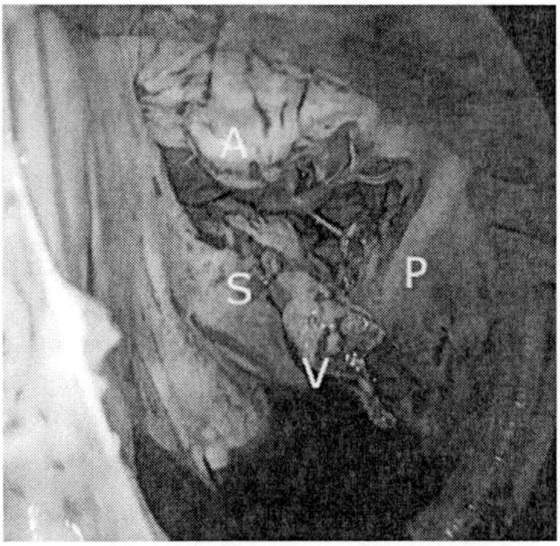

Figure 1. Right Sided Endocarditis in a drug abuser involving the septal leaflet as seen at the time of surgery. The lesion was excised and a bioprosthesis implanted through a minimally invasive right thoracotomy approach A: anterior leaflet; P: posterior leaflet; S: septal leaflet; V: endocarditic vegetation (photo courtesy of G. Bianchi MD PhD, personal archive).

The choice of type of prosthetic valve is dependent on several factors, including age, anticoagulation parameters, sex (woman in child-bearing age), coexistence with another prosthetic valve, history of thromboembolic complications, existence of chronic atrial fibrillation [79]. If a mechanical valve prosthesis should be chosen, a bileaflet with homoaxial flow (e.g., St Jude M, or ON-X) could be the valve of first choice. However, comparative results derived from various studies demonstrate no significant differences concerning the operative mortality, survival rate as well as rate of freedom from reoperation [57, 80, 81]. Finally, in a meta-analysis, Rizzoli et al. showed no survival benefit between a bioprosthetic or a mechanical valve [82].

The management of pacemaker and ICD endocarditis is both medical and surgical, since it systematically requires complete extraction of the device. The reported mortality rates for ICD endocarditis without device extraction ranges from 31 to 66%, compared with 18% in patients in whom the hardware is extracted, followed by prolonged antibiotic therapy [8, 56]. According to Margey et al., among 39 patients suffering from endocarditis, complete device extraction was undertaken in 82%; none had a subsequent relapse, and their mortality rate was 7.4% in contrast to patients managed with partial removal or conservative therapy, relapse occurred in 67% with mortality occurring in 8.4% of them [35]. In pacemaker-dependent patients, a temporary transvenous pacing wire may be implanted to allow at least 7 days until another permanent system is implanted. However, in stable, non-bacteremic patients with no valvular involvement, a new device can probably be implanted earlier. Of note, in about 88–90% of patients undergoing device extraction, removal was performed percutaneously, while only in 10–12% of cases, a median sternotomy and use of extracorporeal circulation was required.

Conclusion

RSIE is a relevant cause of morbidity among IDUs and patients with CIED and indwelling vascular devices. The prognosis of RSIE is usually good and it can be conservatively managed in the majority of cases. However, it can represent a challenge to the cardiac surgeon, due to poor postoperative compliance and high relapse rate in IDUs. Hence, management of RSIE prompts for a multispecialty, tailored approach including cardiologists, cardiac surgeons and infectious disease specialists.

References

[1] Chan P, Ogilby JD, Segal B (1989) Tricuspid valve endocarditis. *Am Heart J* 117:1140–1146.

[2] Frontera JA, Gradon JD (2000) Right-side endocarditis in injection drug users: review of proposed mechanisms of pathogenesis. *Clin Infect Dis* 30:374–379.

[3] del Rìo A, Anguera I, Miró JM, Mont L, Fowler Jr VG, Azqueta M, Mestres CA, Group HCES, others (2003) Surgical treatment of pacemaker and defibrillator lead endocarditis: the impact of electrode lead extraction on outcome. *Chest* 124:1451–1459.

[4] Sohail MR, Uslan DZ, Khan AH, Friedman PA, Hayes DL, Wilson WR, Steckelberg JM, Stoner S, Baddour LM (2007) Management and outcome of permanent pacemaker and implantable cardioverter-defibrillator infections. *J Am Coll Cardiol* 49:1851–1859.

[5] Morokuma H, Minato N, Kamohara K, Minematsu N (2010) Three surgical cases of isolated tricuspid valve infective endocarditis. *Ann Thorac Cardiovasc Surg* 16:134–8.

[6] Alexiou C, Langley SM, Monro JL (1999) Surgery for infective valve endocarditis in children. *Eur J Cardiothorac Surg* 16:653–659.

[7] Musci M, Siniawski H, Pasic M, Grauhan O, Weng Y, Meyer R, Yankah CA, Hetzer R (2007) Surgical treatment of right-sided active infective endocarditis with or without involvement of the left heart: 20-year single center experience. *Eur J Cardiothorac Surg* 32:118–125.

[8] Sohail MR, Uslan DZ, Khan AH, Friedman PA, Hayes DL, Wilson WR, Steckelberg JM, Jenkins SM, Baddour LM (2008) Infective endocarditis complicating permanent pacemaker and implantable cardioverter-defibrillator infection. In: Mayo Clin. Proc. Elsevier, pp 46–53.

[9] Chrissoheris MP, Libertin C, Ali RG, Ghantous A, Bekui A, Donohue T (2009) Endocarditis complicating central venous catheter bloodstream infections: a unique form of health care associated endocarditis. *Clin Cardiol* 32:E48–E54.

[10] Hecht SR, Berger M (1992) Right-sided endocarditis in intravenous drug users: prognostic features in 102 episodes. *Ann Intern Med* 117:560–566.

[11] Moss R, Munt B (2003) Injection drug use and right sided endocarditis. *Heart* 89:577–581.

[12] Grover A, Anand IS, Varma J, Choudhury R, Khattri HN, Sapru RP, Bidwai PS, Wahi PL (1991) Profile of right-sided endocarditis: an Indian experience. *Int J Cardiol* 33:83–88.

[13] Cabell CH, Heidenreich PA, Chu VH, Moore CM, Stryjewski ME, Corey GR, Fowler Jr VG (2004) Increasing rates of cardiac device infections among Medicare beneficiaries: 1990–1999. *Am Heart J* 147:582–586.

[14] Revilla A, López J, Villacorta E, et al. (2008) Isolated right-sided valvular endocarditis in non-intravenous drug users. *Rev Esp Cardiol Engl* Ed 61:1253–1259.

[15] Ruttmann E, Hangler HB, Kilo J, HÖfer D, MÜller LC, Hintringer F, MÜller S, Laufer Gü, Antretter H (2006) Transvenous pacemaker lead removal is safe and effective even in large vegetations: an analysis of 53 cases of pacemaker lead endocarditis. *Pacing Clin Electrophysiol* 29:231–236.

[16] Nori US, Manoharan A, Thornby JI, Yee J, Parasuraman R, Ramanathan V (2006) Mortality risk factors in chronic haemodialysis patients with infective endocarditis. *Nephrol Dial Transplant* 21:2184–2190.

[17] Rankin JS, Milford-Beland S, O'Brien SM, Edwards FH, Peterson ED, Glower DD, Ferguson TB, others (2007) The risk of valve surgery for endocarditis in patients with dialysis-dependent renal failure. *J Heart Valve Dis* 16:617–22.

[18] Habib G, Microbiology E by the ES of C, Diseases (ESCMID) I, et al. (2009) Guidelines on the prevention, diagnosis, and treatment of infective endocarditis (new version 2009) The Task Force on the Prevention, Diagnosis, and Treatment of Infective Endocarditis of the European Society of Cardiology (ESC). *Eur Heart J* 30:2369–2413.

[19] Ellis M, Al-Abdely H, Sandridge A, Greer W, Ventura W (2001) Fungal endocarditis: evidence in the world literature, 1965–1995. *Clin Infect Dis* 32:50–62.

[20] Pierrotti LC, Baddour LM (2002) Fungal Endocarditis, 1995–2000. *Chest* 122:302–310.

[21] Falcone M, Tiseo G, Durante-Mangoni E, et al. (2018) Risk factors and outcomes of endocarditis due to non-HACEK Gram-negative bacilli: data from the Prospective Multicenter Italian Endocarditis Study Cohort. *Antimicrob Agents Chemothe*r 62:e02208–17.

[22] Benenson S, Navon-Venezia S, Carmeli Y, Adler A, Strahilevitz J, Moses AE, Block C (2009) Carbapenem-resistant Klebsiella pneumoniae endocarditis in a young adult: successful treatment with gentamicin and colistin. *Int J Infect Dis* 13:e295–e298.

[23] Iacovelli A, Spaziante M, Al Moghazi S, Giordano A, Ceccarelli G, Venditti M (2018) A challenging case of carbapenemase-producing Klebsiella pneumoniae septic thrombophlebitis and right mural endocarditis successfully treated with ceftazidime/avibactam. *Infection* 46:721–724.

[24] Martin-Davila P, Navas E, Fortún J, Moya JL, Cobo J, Pintado V, Quereda C, Jiménez-Mena M, Moreno S (2005) Analysis of mortality and risk factors associated with native valve endocarditis in drug users: the importance of vegetation size. *Am Heart J* 150:1099–1106.

[25] Nucifora G, Badano L, Hysko F, Allocca G, Gianfagna P, Fioretti P (2007) Pulmonary embolism and fever: when should right-sided infective endocarditis be considered? *Circulation* 115:e173–e176.

[26] Pesanti EL, Smith IM (1979) Infective endocarditis with negative blood cultures: an analysis of 52 cases. *Am J Med* 66:43–50.

[27] Clancy CJ, Nguyen MH (2013) Finding the "missing 50%" of invasive candidiasis: how nonculture diagnostics will improve understanding of disease spectrum and transform patient care. *Clin Infect Dis* 56:1284–1292.

[28] Lamoth F, Cruciani M, Mengoli C, Castagnola E, Lortholary O, Richardson M, Marchetti O (2011) β-Glucan antigenemia assay for

the diagnosis of invasive fungal infections in patients with hematological malignancies: a systematic review and meta-analysis of cohort studies from the Third European Conference on Infections in Leukemia (ECIL-3). *Clin Infect Dis* 54:633–643.

[29] Karageorgopoulos DE, Vouloumanou EK, Ntziora F, Michalopoulos A, Rafailidis PI, Falagas ME (2011) β-D-glucan assay for the diagnosis of invasive fungal infections: a meta-analysis. *Clin Infect Dis* 52:750–770.

[30] He S, Hang JP, Zhang L, Wang F, Zhang DC, Gong F-H (2015) A systematic review and meta-analysis of diagnostic accuracy of serum 1, 3-β-D-glucan for invasive fungal infection: focus on cutoff levels. *J Microbiol Immunol Infect* 48:351–361.

[31] Mikulska M, Calandra T, Sanguinetti M, Poulain D, Viscoli C (2010) The use of mannan antigen and anti-mannan antibodies in the diagnosis of invasive candidiasis: recommendations from the Third European Conference on Infections in Leukemia. *Crit Care* 14:R222

[32] Avni T, Leibovici L, Paul M (2011) PCR diagnosis of invasive candidiasis: systematic review and meta-analysis. *J Clin Microbiol* 49:665–670.

[33] Feuchtner GM, Stolzmann P, Dichtl W, et al. (2009) Multislice computed tomography in infective endocarditis: comparison with transesophageal echocardiography and intraoperative findings. *J Am Coll Cardiol* 53:436–444.

[34] Roman JAS, Vilacosta I (1995) Role of Transesophageal Echocardiography in Right-Sided Endocarditis. *Echocardiography* 12:669–672.

[35] Margey R, McCann H, Blake G, Keelan E, Galvin J, Lynch M, Mahon N, Sugrue D, O'Neill J (2010) Contemporary management of and outcomes from cardiac device related infections. *Eur Eur Pacing Arrhythm Card Electrophysiol J Work Groups Card Pacing Arrhythm Card Cell Electrophysiol Eur Soc Cardiol* 12:64–70.

[36] Habib G, Lancellotti P, Antunes MJ, et al. (2015) 2015 ESC Guidelines for the management of infective endocarditis: The Task Force for the Management of Infective Endocarditis of the European

Society of Cardiology (ESC). Endorsed by: European Association for Cardio-Thoracic Surgery (EACTS), the European Association of Nuclear Medicine (EANM). *Eur Heart J* 36:3075–3128.

[37] Rasmussen RV, Høst U, Arpi M, et al. (2011) Prevalence of infective endocarditis in patients with Staphylococcus aureus bacteraemia: the value of screening with echocardiography. *Eur J Echocardiogr J Work Group Echocardiogr Eur Soc Cardiol* 12:414–420.

[38] Incani A, Hair C, Purnell P, O'Brien DP, Cheng AC, Appelbe A, Athan E (2013) Staphylococcus aureus bacteraemia: evaluation of the role of transoesophageal echocardiography in identifying clinically unsuspected endocarditis. *Eur J Clin Microbiol Infect Dis Off Publ Eur Soc Clin Microbiol* 32:1003–1008.

[39] Berdejo J, Shibayama K, Harada K, Tanaka J, Mihara H, Gurudevan SV, Siegel RJ, Shiota T (2014) Evaluation of vegetation size and its relationship with embolism in infective endocarditis: a real-time 3-dimensional transesophageal echocardiography study. *Circ Cardiovasc Imaging* 7:149–154.

[40] Narducci ML, Pelargonio G, Russo E, et al. (2013) Usefulness of intracardiac echocardiography for the diagnosis of cardiovascular implantable electronic device-related endocarditis. *J Am Coll Cardiol* 61:1398–1405.

[41] Saby L, Laas O, Habib G, et al. (2013) Positron emission tomography/computed tomography for diagnosis of prosthetic valve endocarditis: increased valvular 18F-fluorodeoxyglucose uptake as a novel major criterion. *J Am Coll Cardiol* 61:2374–2382.

[42] Erba PA, Conti U, Lazzeri E, et al. (2012) Added value of 99mTc-HMPAO-labeled leukocyte SPECT/CT in the characterization and management of patients with infectious endocarditis. *J Nucl Med Off Publ Soc Nucl Me*d 53:1235–1243.

[43] Rouzet F, Chequer R, Benali K, Lepage L, Ghodbane W, Duval X, Iung B, Vahanian A, Le Guludec D, Hyafil F (2014) Respective performance of 18F-FDG PET and radiolabeled leukocyte scintigraphy for the diagnosis of prosthetic valve endocarditis. *J Nucl Med Off Publ Soc Nucl Med* 55:1980–1985.

[44] McDanel JS, Roghmann M-C, Perencevich EN, et al. (2017) Comparative Effectiveness of Cefazolin Versus Nafcillin or Oxacillin for Treatment of Methicillin-Susceptible Staphylococcus aureus Infections Complicated by Bacteremia: *A Nationwide Cohort Study. Clin Infect Dis Off Publ Infect Dis Soc Am* 65:100–106.

[45] Buchholtz K, Larsen CT, Schaadt B, Hassager C, Bruun NE (2011) Once versus twice daily gentamicin dosing for infective endocarditis: a randomized clinical trial. *Cardiology* 119:65–71.

[46] Miro' JM, García-de-la-Mària C, Armero Y, et al. (2009) Addition of gentamicin or rifampin does not enhance the effectiveness of daptomycin in treatment of experimental endocarditis due to methicillin-resistant Staphylococcus aureus. *Antimicrob Agents Chemother* 53:4172–4177.

[47] Fernández-Hidalgo N, Almirante B, Gavaldà J, et al. (2013) Ampicillin plus ceftriaxone is as effective as ampicillin plus gentamicin for treating enterococcus faecalis infective endocarditis. *Clin Infect Dis Off Publ Infect Dis Soc Am* 56:1261–1268.

[48] White RL, Burgess DS, Manduru M, Bosso JA (1996) Comparison of three different in vitro methods of detecting synergy: time-kill, checkerboard, and E test. *Antimicrob Agents Chemother* 40:1914–1918.

[49] Boumis E, Gesu G, Menichetti F, et al. (2010) Consensus document on controversial issues in the diagnosis and treatment of bloodstream infections and endocarditis. *Int J Infect Dis* IJID Off Publ Int Soc Infect Dis 14 Suppl 4:S23-38.

[50] Pappas PG, Kauffman CA, Andes DR, et al. (2016) Executive Summary: Clinical Practice Guideline for the Management of Candidiasis: 2016 Update by the Infectious Diseases Society of America. *Clin Infect Dis Off Publ Infect Dis Soc Am* 62:409–417.

[51] Akinosoglou K, Apostolakis E, Koutsogiannis N, Leivaditis V, Gogos CA (2012) Right-sided infective endocarditis: surgical management. *Eur J Cardio-Thorac Surg Off J Eur Assoc Cardio-Thorac Surg* 42:470–479.

[52] Lowes JA, Hamer J, Williams G, Houang E, Tabaqchali S, Shaw EJ, Hill IM, Rees GM (1980) 10 Years of infective endocarditis at St. Bartholomew's Hospital: analysis of clinical features and treatment in relation to prognosis and mortality. *Lancet Lond Engl* 1:133–136.

[53] Bayer AS, Blomquist IK, Bello E, Chiu CY, Ward JI, Ginzton LE (1988) Tricuspid valve endocarditis due to Staphylococcus aureus. Correlation of two-dimensional echocardiography with clinical outcome. *Chest* 93:247–253.

[54] Gottardi R, Bialy J, Devyatko E, Tschernich H, Czerny M, Wolner E, Seitelberger R (2007) Midterm follow-up of tricuspid valve reconstruction due to active infective endocarditis. *Ann Thorac Surg* 84:1943–1948.

[55] Head SJ, Mokhles MM, Osnabrugge RLJ, Bogers AJJC, Kappetein AP (2011) Surgery in current therapy for infective endocarditis. *Vasc Health Risk Manag* 7:255–263.

[56] Cacoub P, Leprince P, Nataf P, Hausfater P, Dorent R, Wechsler B, Bors V, Pavie A, Piette JC, Gandjbakhch I (1998) Pacemaker infective endocarditis. *Am J Cardiol* 82:480–484.

[57] Moon MR, Stinson EB, Miller DC (1997) Surgical treatment of endocarditis. *Prog Cardiovasc Dis* 40:239–264.

[58] Remadi JP, Habib G, Nadji G, Brahim A, Thuny F, Casalta JP, Peltier M, Tribouilloy C (2007) Predictors of death and impact of surgery in Staphylococcus aureus infective endocarditis. *Ann Thorac* Surg 83:1295–1302.

[59] Rubinstein E, Lang R (1995) Fungal endocarditis. *Eur Heart J* 16 Suppl B:84–89.

[60] Morpeth S, Murdoch D, Cabell CH, et al. (2007) Non-HACEK gram-negative bacillus endocarditis. *Ann Intern Med* 147:829–835.

[61] Jacobs F, Abramowicz D, Vereerstraeten P, Le Clerc JL, Zech F, Thys JP (1990) Brucella endocarditis: the role of combined medical and surgical treatment. *Rev Infect Dis* 12:740–744.

[62] Tasdemir K, Kaya MG, Mavili E, Gunebakmaz O, Ozbek A, Sarli B, Yarlioglues M, Emirogullari N (2010) Surgical approach to the

management of Brucella endocarditis. *Eur J Cardio-Thorac Surg Off J Eur Assoc Cardio-Thorac Surg* 37:1021–1024.
[63] Horstkotte D, Follath F, Gutschik E, et al. (2004) Guidelines on prevention, diagnosis and treatment of infective endocarditis executive summary; the task force on infective endocarditis of the European society of cardiology. *Eur Heart J* 25:267–276.
[64] Frater RW (1990) Surgical management of endocarditis in drug addicts and long-term results. *J Card Surg* 5:63–67.
[65] DiNubile M (1987) Surgery for addiction-related tricuspid valve endocarditis: caveat emptor. *Am J Med* 82:811–813.
[66] Chang B-C, Lim S-H, Yi G, Hong YS, Lee S, Yoo K-J, Kang MS, Cho BK (2006) Long-term clinical results of tricuspid valve replacement. *Ann Thorac Surg* 81:1317–1324.
[67] Chang HW, Jeong DS, Cho YH, Sung K, Kim WS, Lee YT, Park PW (2017) Tricuspid Valve Replacement vs. Repair in Severe Tricuspid Regurgitation. *Circ J* 81:330–338.
[68] Lange R, Piazza N, Günther T (2017) Tricuspid valve regurgitation: Indications and operative techniques. Herz 42:653–661.
[69] Yee ES, Khonsari S (1989) Right-sided infective endocarditis: valvuloplasty, valvectomy or replacement. *J Cardiovasc Surg* (Torino) 30:744–748.
[70] Allen MD, Slachman F, Eddy AC, Cohen D, Otto CM, Pearlman AS (1991) Tricuspid valve repair for tricuspid valve endocarditis: tricuspid valve "recycling." *Ann Thorac Surg* 51:593–598.
[71] Lange R, De Simone R, Bauernschmitt R, Tanzeem A, Schmidt C, Hagl S (1996) Tricuspid valve reconstruction, a treatment option in acute endocarditis. *Eur J Cardio-Thorac Surg Off J Eur Assoc Cardio-Thorac Surg* 10:320–326.
[72] Romano G, Carozza A, Della Corte A, De Santo LS, Amarelli C, Torella M, De Feo M, Cerasuolo F, Cotrufo M (2004) Native versus primary prosthetic valve endocarditis: comparison of clinical features and long-term outcome in 353 patients. *J Heart Valve Dis* 13:200–208; discussion 208-209.

[73] Miro' JM, del Río A, Mestres CA (2003) Infective endocarditis and cardiac surgery in intravenous drug abusers and HIV-1 infected patients. *Cardiol Clin* 21:167–184, v–vi.

[74] Kaiser SP, Melby SJ, Zierer A, Schuessler RB, Moon MR, Moazami N, Pasque MK, Huddleston C, Damiano RJ, Lawton JS (2007) Long-term outcomes in valve replacement surgery for infective endocarditis. *Ann Thorac Surg* 83:30–35.

[75] Al-Ebrahim KE (2010) Tricuspid valve replacement is an unfavourable operation. *Eur J Cardio-Thorac Surg Off J Eur Assoc Cardio-Thorac Surg* 38:115.

[76] Guenther T, Noebauer C, Mazzitelli D, Busch R, Tassani-Prell P, Lange R (2008) Tricuspid valve surgery: a thirty-year assessment of early and late outcome. *Eur J Cardio-Thorac Surg Off J Eur Assoc Cardio-Thorac Surg* 34:402–409; discussion 409.

[77] Singh SK, Tang GH, Maganti MD, Armstrong S, Williams WG, David TE, Borger MA (2006) Midterm outcomes of tricuspid valve repair versus replacement for organic tricuspid disease. *Ann Thorac Surg* 82:1735–1741.

[78] Moraca RJ, Moon MR, Lawton JS, Guthrie TJ, Aubuchon KA, Moazami N, Pasque MK, Damiano RJ (2009) Outcomes of tricuspid valve repair and replacement: a propensity analysis. *Ann Thorac Surg* 87:83–88; discussion 88-89.

[79] Shemin R (2008) Tricuspid valve disease. In: Cohn LH (ed) *Card. Surg. Adult* 3rd Edn. McGraw-Hill, New York, Chicago, San Francisco, pp 1118–22.

[80] Ratnatunga CP, Edwards MB, Dore CJ, Taylor KM (1998) Tricuspid valve replacement: UK Heart Valve Registry mid-term results comparing mechanical and biological prostheses. *Ann Thorac Surg* 66:1940–1947.

[81] Kaplan M, Kut MS, Demirtas MM, Cimen S, Ozler A (2002) Prosthetic replacement of tricuspid valve: bioprosthetic or mechanical. *Ann Thorac Surg* 73:467–473.

[82] Rizzoli G, Vendramin I, Nesseris G, Bottio T, Guglielmi C, Schiavon L (2004) Biological or mechanical prostheses in tricuspid position? A meta-analysis of intra-institutional results. *Ann Thorac Surg* 77:1607–1614.

In: The Rediscovered Tricuspid Valve ISBN: 978-1-53616-098-7
Editor: Giacomo Bianchi

Chapter 8

TRICUSPID VALVE DISEASE IN ADULTS WITH CONGENITAL HEART DISEASE IN NATURAL OR MODIFIED HISTORY

Elisa Barberi[1,*], MD and Vitali Pak[2], MD
[1]Pediatric Intensive Care Unit, Ospedale del Cuore,
Fondazione Toscana "G. Monasterio", Massa, Italy
[2]Department of Pediatric Cardiac Surgery, Ospedale del Cuore,
Fondazione Toscana "G. Monasterio", Massa, Italy

ABSTRACT

Improved medical and surgical management of congenital heart disease has led to increased survival of these patients into adulthood. Currently, the number of congenital heart disease grown-up patients has exceeded that of the paediatric population with congenital heart defects. These patients need specialized and multidisciplinary care. Particularly in these patients the tricuspid valve takes on great importance, since in some diseases it is the only atrioventricular valve. The approach to the tricuspid valve in the adult congenital can therefore not ignore the knowledge of

* Corresponding Author's E-mail: elisa.barberi@ftgm.it.

how surgery determines a change in the natural history of the underlying disease, and which non-invasive and invasive techniques can be used to quantify the severity. By integrating these results, the clinician and the surgeon are called upon to plan the most suitable therapeutic path, knowing the medical and surgical treatment options.

Keywords: Tricuspid valve, ACHD, CHD, GUCH

Introduction

Improved medical and surgical care of congenital heart disease patients increased survival into adulthood from 15% in the 1960s to over 85% in the current era. As a consequence, the number of adults with congenital heart disease (ACHD) will inevitably increase, and recent data affirm that in Europe, we are actually faced with an estimated patient population of 2.3 million. The number of ACHD has already exceeded that of the pediatric population with congenital heart disease (CHD) [1].

Although initially considered to be cured, the majority of them continue to need specialized follow-up because they require re-do interventions or are at increased risk of cardiovascular complications and premature death. These patients, particularly the adults with moderate and highly complex CHD, can be very difficult to manage, and should be treated in few experienced and specialized 'grown-up congenital heart disease' (GUCH) units, concentrating resources, patients, funding, and professional experiences [2].

Tricuspid Valve in ACHD

The tricuspid valve (TV) is often called the "forgotten valve" or "lost valve" [3] because it is relatively understudied compared to the other cardiac valves [4, 5]. Tricuspid valve disease is a frequent primary and secondary issue in adult congenital heart disease (ACHD), although its incidence has not been well defined [6]. It has received less attention in terms of research or guidelines. Indications for surgical intervention, and methods of approach and repair, are not uniform across institutions. In the last decade progress has been made in comprehension the pathology of the tricuspid valve, especially tricuspid regurgitation. A greater understanding of the contribution of this injury on symptoms, morbidity and mortality is derived from the acquired pathology. Imaging of the tricuspid valve is often required and is complex and multimodality [7]. In patients with congenital heart defects, the tricuspid valve often assumes particular importance. In fact, in patients with hypoplastic left heart syndrome, it is the only functional atrioventricular valve. In other defects such as pulmonary atresia with intact ventricular septum, tricuspid valve function can be the limiting factor for a successful surgical outcome. Long-term outcomes after a Mustard or Senning operation for transposition of the great arteries depend largely on how well the tricuspid valve functions as the systemic atrioventricular valve.

More rigorous and in-depht studies will be needed to understand the extent of the problem in the ACHD population.

EMBRIOLOGY AND ANATOMY OF THE TRICUSPID VALVE

The septation of atria and ventricles in the fetal circulation is followed by formation of endocardial cushions at the crux of the heart. The atrio-ventricular (AV) valves develop subsequently. Prior to septation the right atrium communicates directly into the cavity of the left ventricle. The ventricle septation communicates right atrium to the right ventricle and subsequently the TV leaflets and their tension apparatus develops. The septal leaflet is formed from the muscular ventricular septum together with postero-inferior endocardial cushions. This may provide an explanation for the septal leaflets participating in spontaneous closure of a small perimembranous ventricular septal defect in childhood. The architecture of the two valve is intimately tied to the corresponding ventricles. These relationships are emphasized in the congenitally corrected transposition of the great arteries (ccTGA) with functionally intact circulation, such that the anatomic right ventricle becomes the systemic ventricle and anatomic left ventricle becomes the pulmonary ventricle. The corresponding AV valves are transposed along with ventricles. Since the formation of AV cushions at the crux of the heart are central to distinctive anatomy of the two AV valves, the congenital absence of AV cushions, partial or complete, result in striking abnormalities of the two AV valves [8].

The TV is the right-sided AV valve and it is most caudally located and has largest orifice among the four intracardiac valves. It functions as a unidirectional valve permitting systemic venous blood flow from right atrium, and hence from the two vena cava and the coronary sinus, to the right ventricle during diastole and prevents backflow during systole. The cyclical opening and closure of the valve, as well as the right atrial contraction, provides the pulsatile nature of vena cava flow. Since the right ventricle is a low-pressure chamber facing a low-resistance pulmonary circulation, the pressure difference from right ventricle to right atrium in systole is small [9].

The TV apparatus is composed of the anulus, the leaflets, the chordae and papillary muscles. The anulus is oval in shape and is displaced more toward the apex than in the mitral valve. It assumes a more circular shape on dilatation. The TV has three leaflets: anterior, septal and posterior, the anterior being the largest and septal being the smallest. The tendinous chords are attached to the ventricle surface of the leaflets or the free edges of the leaflets to the papillary muscle supporting the leaflet. There are three sets of papillary muscles, each set being composed of up to three muscles. Several important anatomic structures are closely related to the TV. The triangle of Koch sits superiorly to the septal leaflet and is made up of the coronary sinus ostium at its base, the tendon of Todaro and the septal leaflet of the TV. At its apex lies the AV node, which is susceptible to damage during surgery. Anterior to this structure lies the central fibrous body, penetrated by the His bundle, and further anterior lies the membranous septum. The mitral anulus is leftward of the tricuspid anulus. The aortic valve lies in the space between the two AV valves anteriorly [10].

Etiology of Tricuspid Valve Disease

The TV disease is generally classified as primary or intrinsic valve pathology or secondary or functional valve dysfunction.

The primary valve disease occurs when there is a damage to the tricuspid leaflets, chordae, papillary muscles, or anulus, independent of right ventricular dysfunction or pulmonary hypertension. Over time, severe tricuspid regurgitation that is initially non-functional, can led into functional tricuspid regurgitation, related to progressive right ventricular dysfunction [11].

The secondary or functional TV disease results from the factors that generally lead to tricuspid anular dilatation commonly from left heart disease and resulting right ventricle hypertension, dilatation and dysfunction. More than 75% of severe tricuspid regurgitation is classified as functional [12]. Functional TR carries a significant adverse prognosis in acquired heart disease [13, 14]. Whether this adverse prognosis can be applied in congenital heart disease remains to be proved. Functional TR in CHD may occur in many lesions in which there is abnormal preload or afterload affecting the RV, such as atrial septal defect (ASD), anomalous pulmonary venous return, pulmonary regurgitation, pulmonary hypertension, and in the failing systemic RV [15].

Tricuspid Valve Disease in ACHD

The tricuspid valve disease in ACHD occurs essentially in this spectrum of pathologies:

Patients with Ebstein's Anomaly

Ebstein's anomaly accounts for less than 1% of CHD and is a complex and heterogeneous form of cardiac disease characterized by malformation and apical displacement of the TV leaflets toward the apex of the RV. While the anulus remains in the normal position, the attachments of the septal and posterior leaflets are rotationally displaced from the AV ring, and the anterior leaflet is tipically elongated and sail-like. There is subsequent variable thinning of the wall of the "atrialized" RV along with redundancy and tethering of the anterior leaflet of the TV [16]. The clinical manifestations of Ebstein's anomaly depend largely on the degree of severity of the TV displacement and the resultant physiologic effect. RV function becomes regurgitant, resulting in decreased forward flow through the pulmonary valve. The combined right atrium and atrialized RV becomes dilated with right-to-left shunt across interatrial septum. Ebstein's anomaly is the only CHD that has a range of clinical presentations from the severely symptomatic neonate to an asymptomatic adult. In the adult the most common initial symptom is exercise intolerance and the severity of clinical signs depends on the degree of displacement of TV leaflets [17].

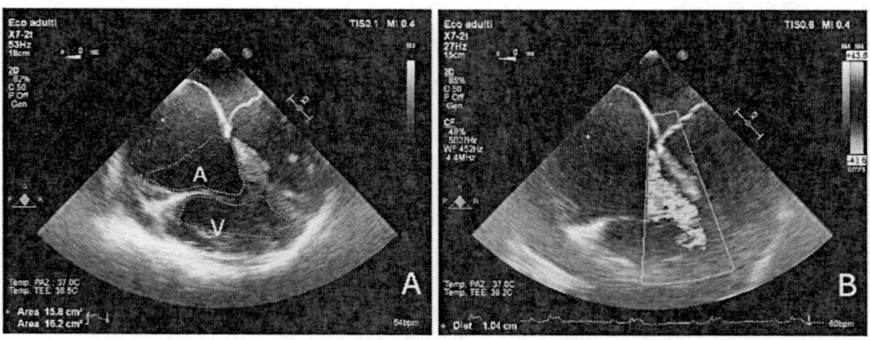

Figure 1. Ebstein's anomaly in a 32-year old patient in natural history. Panel A: atrialized (A) portion of the right ventricle is bigger than the right ventricle itself (B). Panel B: tricuspid valve regurgitation (Vena Contracta width is shown) indicating severe TR.

Several factors play a part: TR, ventricular dysfunction, right-to-left shunt, reduced cardiac output. With increased age, adults with Ebstein's anomaly present with arrythmias and in those patients with patent foramen ovale, risk of embolisation, brain abscess and sudden death [18, 19].

Tricuspid Valve Disease Caused by Previous Interventions

In the atrio-ventricular septal defect the right-sided AV valve can occasionally be left with varying degrees of stenosis and regurgitation after repair. In the repair of the perimembranous ventricular septal defect, the septal leaflet of the TV has attachments to the septum and these can be damaged during repair, leading to significant TR. Patients with repaired Tetralogy of Fallot and pulmonary stenosis are commonly left with severe pulmonary regurgitation. This regurgitation can lead to RV dilatation and dysfunction over time. Secondary TR can result from this. ACHD usually present heart block or ventricular arrhythmias and necessitate placement of pacemakers or ICDs. The ventricular lead can damage leaflet perforation, laceration or scarring/adhesion to the lead. In patients with pulmonary atresia with intact ventricular septum, as part of biventricular repair, significant pulmonary regurgitation often occurs. This condition can lead to dilatation of the right ventricle which is connected with a TV hypoplastic [6].

Systemic Right Ventricle in Congenitally Corrected Transposition of the Great Arteries (ccTGA) or Transposition of the Great Arteries (D-TGA) after Mustard/Senning Operation and Hypoplastic Left Heart Syndrome (HLHS).

TR can occur in CCTGA, in which dysplasia of the tricuspid valve (sharing some features with Ebstein anomaly) is a common finding. Tricuspid valve replacement is recommended in this situation if significant AV valve regurgitation is appreciated, and may prevent deterioration in systemic RV function over time. In contrast with this, TR in D-TGA after Mustard or Senning operation is often secondary. Akin to functional mitral regurgitation, tricuspid valve replacement is not advised if there is significant dysfunction of the systemic RV. TR is a risk factor for mortality in patients with HLHS. Up to 25% of patients after Norwood operation require surgery for TR. The tricuspid valve may be regurgitant in these patients because of systemic RV dysfunction or intrinsic abnormalities of the tricuspid valve, including dysplasia, prolapse, and increased/ decreased number of leaflets [20].

Functional Tricuspid Valve Disease in ACHD

Functional TV disease in ACHD is related to RV dilation/dysfunction, usually as a consequence of chronic RV volume overloading. This is an emerging problem by the fact that ACHD represents a growing patient population but still often underestimated. For example, a chronic left-to-right shunting in an atrial septal defect can lead to long-term volume overload of RV. When this overload causes anular dilatation or dysfunction, secondary TR can ensue.

Functional TR is associated with chronic RV volume overloading typically for example in patients with large atrial septal defect or pulmonary valve regurgitation despite the increasing number of interventional procedures available in the catheterisation lab. The tricuspid anulus is a component of both the TV and the RV. Dilatation of the tricuspid anulus is only possible in the anteroposterior aspects which correspond to the free wall of the right ventricle. In adults with ASD or chronic pulmonary valve regurgitation, RV dilatation causes left-sided septal bulging and the consequence is the anular dilatation and leaflet tethering of the TV. TR will be moderate to severe.

Pulmonary hypertension by itself does not usually cause TR, but, when RV dilatation and dysfunction develop, secondary TR can result.

The number of patients with functional TR will increase in the years as will the number with ACHD. Today, although operations in ACHD have become frequent, the surgical treatment is rarely reported. The concept that functional TR does not disappear when the primary lesion has been corrected should be more accepted, and consequently a more aggressive approach should be considered when treating these patients. Surgery to correct functional TR can be performed at low risk. Generally, a tricuspid valve repair, however, a substitution can be easily performed, and these patients generally benefit from significant clinical improvement [21–26].

CLINICAL PRESENTATIONS OF THE ADULT PATIENT WITH TRICUSPID VALVE DISEASE

Symptoms

Patients with tricuspid valve disease commonly present late in their disease. They present lack of energy and poor exercise capacity. One of the main difficulties in patients with ACHD is that they often have other comorbidities that may contribute to exercise intolerance and are typical of the GUCH patient: ventricular dysfunction, associated valvular disease, univentricular physiology, right-to-left shunting with cyanosis, arrhythmia requiring pacemakers and causes of non-cardiac limitation, such as restrictive lung disease, obesity and general frailty. Other typical features of the tricuspid pathology are abdominal fullness caused by hepatic and intestinal venous distension and subsequent ascites. As the disease progresses, anorexia occurs leading to malnutrition and loss of muscle and fat mass. Cachexia can be masked by massive fluid overload. Swelling and edema of the legs occur [27].

Physical Signs

Tricuspid stenosis results in characteristic changes in the jugular venous pulse. The liver is enlarged and is pulsatile in presystole. Auscultation reveals a low-to medium-itched diastolic rumble with inspiration accentuation. Tricuspid regurgitation results in the jugular venous pulse exhibiting a prominent C-V wave or systolic wave. The liver shows systolic pulsations, is enlarged and is often tender. The cardiac auscultation reveals a soft early or holosystolic murmur, which is augmented with inspiratory effort [28].

Non-Invasive and Invasive Diagnostic Tools

In the electrocardiogram there are no specific markers of TV disease, only right ventricle hypertrophy and right atrial enlargement with prominent P-waves. Palpitations are frequent, mostly caused by supraventricular arrhythmia. The commonest arrhythmic complication is atrial flutter, or, in Ebstein anomaly the Wolff-Parkinson-White syndrome, which occurs in approximately 25% [29].

In the chest X-ray cardiomegaly associated with prominent right heart borders may be noted.

A systematic approach to examing the TV by echocardiography should be utilized. This involves evaluating the size of the right-sided cardiac chambers, motion of the interventricular septum and obtaining Doppler parameters and color imaging, in at least 2 orthogonal planes wherever possible. The size of the inferior vena cava (IVC) and response to respiration as well as hepatic vein flow pattern helps evaluate right atrial pressure and adaptations to volume overload.

The AHA/ACC guidelines for assessment of TR [30, 31] utilize central jet area, continuous wave Doppler (CWD) jet density and contour, hepatic vein flow and the hemodynamic consequences of TR on RV/RA/IVC size and RV function. The American Society of Echocardiography (ASE) and the European Association of Echocardiography (EAE) both recommend very similar parameters. The most commonly assessment of the TV is with transthoracic (TTE) imaging. The main views for visualization of the TV are the parasternal LAX, apical four chamber and subcostal views, however none of these windows can image all leaflets of the TV simultaneousl. The current AHA/ACC guideline defines the "tricuspid annular dilation", at which TV repair should be considered as > 40 mm or > 21 mm/m^2, and is based on a TTE 4 chamber measure. TTE is important in assessing the severity of TR and RVSP as the images are obtained in a conscious patient with normal resting hemodynamics. A baseline TTE study is also used to elucidate the etiology of TR, measure the size of right-sided chambers and the IVC, assess RV systolic function, and characterize any associated left sided disease. A comprehensive intraoperative 2D transesophageal echocardiography (TEE) examination remains important. Such a study can investigate for additional findings that may have been missed on TTE and can assist in operative planning and surgical decision making. The altered loading conditions of general anesthesia will change the appearance of TR, generally making it appear less severe. The favorable location of the TEE transducer, close to the heart, allows for higher resolution imaging than with TTE with improved delineation of anatomical structures.

Cardiac catheterization and selective angiography were used prior to the advent of diagnostic echocardiography.

In the recent years, cardiac magnetic resonance imaging has become the gold standard in assessment of right ventricular volumes and function. This modality also allow reliable serial imaging to assess changes in right ventricular size and volume to follow TV disease over time [32].

Cardiac computed tomography can be used as an alternative with newer techniques leading to reduced radiation dose.

Management of the Adult Patient with Tricuspid Valve Disease

Non-Surgical Therapy

The evaluation and the severity of the tricuspid valve disease is necessary to define its impact. It is important to determine the eziology and the clinical presentation of the patient. In an overall approach we should manage factors like arrhythmia, pulmonary hypertension, left-sided heart disease, valvular disease, infection [33].

The non-surgical therapy must improve the clinical status in terms of edema, shortness of breath, abdominal swelling, ascite. Diuretics control the volume overload: loop diuretics are the first used and the addition of thiazide diuretics can sometimes be warranted. Inotropic support can be useful in right ventricular dysfunction and, in case of pulmonary hypertension, vasodilators are appropriate. Antiarrhythmics should be considered to control supraventricular arrhythmias or eventually ablation. Valve-in-valve replacement to TV is considered when there is a bioprosthetic valve dysfunction.

Surgical Therapy

In ACHD an enormous variability of the disorders of the tricuspid valve and a frequently additional component of functional tricuspid valve are present. The patient's clinical status and the cause of the tricuspid valve abnormality usually determine the appropriate therapeutic strategy.

Table 1. ACC/AHA guidelines for Adults with Congenital Heart Disease

CLASS I 1. Tricuspid valve repair is beneficial for severe TR in patients with MV disease requiring MV surgery. *(Level of Evidence: B)* CLASS IIa • Tricuspid valve replacement or annuloplasty is reasonable for severe primary TR when symptomatic. *(Level of Evidence: C)* • Tricuspid valve replacement is reasonable for severe TR secondary to diseased/abnormal tricuspid valve leaflets not amenable to annuloplasty or repair. *(Level of Evidence: C)* CLASS IIb • Tricuspid annuloplasty may be considered for less than severe TR in patients undergoing MV surgery when there is pulmonary hypertension or tricuspid annular dilatation. *(Level of Evidence: C)* CLASS III • Tricuspid valve replacement or annuloplasty is not indicated in asymptomatic patients with TR whose pulmonary artery systolic pressure is less than 60 mm Hg in the presence of a normal MV. *(Level of Evidence: C)* • Tricuspid valve replacement or annuloplasty is not indicated in patients with mild primary TR. *(Level of Evidence: C)*

This means we should know very well the types of surgeries, their risks and potential long-term outcomes. The type of surgery must be tailored to the underlying disorder but the timing of surgical intervention remains controversial. This controversy has diminished since the advent of 2D and Doppler echocardiography. Intraoperative TEE allows refinement.

The American College of Cardiology (ACC) and the American Heart Association (AHA) ACHD care guidelines mention the tricuspid valve when addressing certain surgical indications [30, 34] (Table 1).

Tricuspid Valve Repair and Tricuspid Valve Replacement

Correction of annular dilatation can be achieved with a variety of annuloplasty methods. The techniques for reducing the annular dimensions include [33, 35, 36]:

- Suture-based techniques include Kay and De Vega annuloplasty. These have a low cost, a low risk of complication and a moderate duration. De Vega annuloplasty involves a wider suture line than Kay annuloplasty and is believed to be more effective.
- Annuloplasty rings provide a more rigid support. They can be partial or full. Partial annuloplasty rings have the advantage of leaving an area around the location of the AV node free of sutures to avoid AV block. However, full annuloplasty rings can be sewn into the septal leaflet to avoid suturing directly into the anulus in the location of the AV node.
- Commissural or cleft closure for areas of commissural/cleft leak.
- Leaflet repair: perforations/fenestrations can be repaired with direct suturing or a patch of autologous or glutaraldehyde-treated pericardium.
- Cusp augmentation: autologous pericardium or the use of prosthetic materials has been used to increase the length of the anterior leaflet or other leaflets in order to increase the degree of coaptation.
- Clover technique.

When satisfactory repair cannot be achieved, tricuspid valve replacement is appropriate. Currently most patients are referred for bioprosthetic tricuspid valve replacement given the significant risk of thrombosis associated with a mechanical valve in this position.

Given the unusual anatomy in Ebstein disorder, surgical options are considered when a patient is symptomatic, cyanotic, in the presence of a paradoxical embolism, progressive cardiomegaly on chest X-ray, progressive RV dilation and may be considered with arrhythmias that are not amenable to percutaneous treatment [37–39]. Due to the relative low risk of surgery in experienced centers, older patients with Ebstein's anomaly have undergone surgery with good outcomes. Da Silva et al. proposed the frequently performed "cone reconstruction" procedure in 2004. In this procedure, the anterior tricuspid valve leaflet is rotated clockwise to form a cone shape, and the base of this cone is sutured to the true tricuspid valve annulus. If needed, plication, or resection of the atrialized right ventricular tissue, is also performed. If repair is not possible, then the tricuspid valve is replaced with a bioprosthetic valve. If present, concomitant procedures such as ASD or PFO closure and/or arrhythmia (MAZE, WPW) ablation are performed. In those patients whose right ventricles are not able to support the pulmonary circulation, bidirectional cavopulmonary anastomosis is considered [40, 41].

In the case of D-TGA or CCTGA the onset of TV disease may be delayed and related to systemic right ventricle. In general, replacement is preferable rather than valve repair to reduce the risk of reoperation. Pulmonary artery banding to restore the crescent shape of the RV was sustained in the past, but the risk of left ventricular failure is high [42].

In the AV septal defect there are often clefts that require primary closure. Associated annular dilatation may require annuloplasty. Valve replacement is rarely required.

A combined arrhythymia surgery like right atial maze or single ablation line across the cavotricuspid isthmus can be appropriate.

Conclusion

Further research on the description of the frequency, severity and results of the disease in ACHD, better ways to quantitatively define intervention times, and the definitive role of earlier and more aggressive surgical and interventional approaches are desirable.

References

[1] Giamberti A, Varrica A, Pomè G, Micheletti A, Negura D, Ranucci M, Carminati M, Frigiola A, Chessa M (2016) The care for adults with congenital heart disease: Organization and function of a grown-up congenital heart disease unit. *Eur Heart J Suppl* 18:E15–E18.

[2] Warnes CA, Williams RG, Bashore TM, et al. (2008) ACC/AHA 2008 Guidelines for the Management of Adults with Congenital Heart Disease: a report of the American College of Cardiology/American Heart Association Task Force on Practice Guidelines (writing committee to develop guidelines on the management of adults with congenital heart disease). *Circulation* 118:e714-833.

[3] Giamberti A, Chessa M (eds) (2014) *The Tricuspid Valve in Congenital Heart Disease.* doi: 10.1007/978-88-470-5400-4.

[4] Tager R, Skudicky D, Mueller U, Essop R, Hammond G, Sareli P (1998) Long-term follow-up of rheumatic patients undergoing left-sided valve replacement with tricuspid annuloplasty—validity of preoperative echocardiographic criteria in the decision to perform tricuspid annuloplasty. *Am J Cardiol* 81:1013–1016.

[5] Bruce CJ, Connolly HM (2009) Right-Sided Valve Disease Deserves a Little More Respect. *Circulation* 119:2726–2734.

[6] Said SM, Burkhart HM, Dearani JA (2012) Surgical Management of Congenital (Non-Ebstein) Tricuspid Valve Regurgitation. *Semin Thorac Cardiovasc Surg Pediatr Card Surg Annu* 15:46–60.

[7] Davlouros PA (2006) The right ventricle in congenital heart disease. *Heart* 92:i27–i38.

[8] Anderson RH (2003) Development of the heart: (2) Septation of the atriums and ventricles. *Heart* 89:949–958.

[9] Shah PM, Raney AA (2008) Tricuspid Valve Disease. *Curr Probl Cardiol* 33:47–84.

[10] Huttin O, Voilliot D, Mandry D, Venner C, Juillière Y, Selton-Suty C (2016) All you need to know about the tricuspid valve: tricuspid valve imaging and tricuspid regurgitation analysis. *Arch Cardiovasc Dis* 109:67–80.

[11] Beckhoff F, Alushi B, Jung C, Navarese E, Franz M, Kretzschmar D, Wernly B, Lichtenauer M, Lauten A (2018) Tricuspid Regurgitation – Medical Management and Evolving Interventional Concepts. *Front Cardiovasc Med.* doi: 10.3389/fcvm.2018.00049.

[12] Mas PT, Rodríguez-Palomares JF, Antunes MJ (2015) Secondary tricuspid valve regurgitation: A forgotten entity. *Heart* 101:1840–1848.

[13] Sagie A, Schwammenthal E, Palacios IF, King ME, Leavitt M, Freitas N, Weyman AE, Levine RA (1994) Significant tricuspid regurgitation does not resolve after percutaneous balloon mitral valvotomy. *J Thorac Cardiovasc Surg* 108:727–735.

[14] Koelling TM, Aaronson KD, Cody RJ, Bach DS, Armstrong WF (2002) Prognostic significance of mitral regurgitation and tricuspid regurgitation in patients with left ventricular systolic dysfunction. *Am Heart J* 144:524–529.

[15] Braunwald NS, Ross JR J, Morrow AG (1967) Conservative management of tricuspid regurgitation in patients undergoing mitral valve replacement. *Circulation* 35:I–63.

[16] Waldmann V, Khairy P (2018) Ventricular arrhythmias and sudden death in patients with Ebstein anomaly: insights from a retrospective cohort study. *J Thorac Dis* 10:S2172–S2175.

[17] Lewin MB, Stout KK (2012) *Echocardiography in Congenital Heart Disease*, 1st ed. Saunders.

[18] Safi LM, Liberthson RR, Bhatt A (2016) Current Management of Ebstein's Anomaly in the Adult. *Curr Treat Options Cardiovasc Med.* doi: 10.1007/s11936-016-0478-2.

[19] Holst KA, Dearani JA, Said S, Pike RB, Connolly HM, Cannon BC, Sessions KL, O\textquotesingleByrne MM, O'Leary PW (2018) Improving Results of Surgery for Ebstein Anomaly: Where Are We After 235 Cone Repairs? *Ann Thorac Surg* 105:160–168.

[20] Kron IL, Roeser ME (2017) Management of Ebstein's anomaly. *Ann Cardiothorac Surg* 6:266–269.

[21] Mangieri A, Montalto C, Pagnesi M, Jabbour RJ, Rodés-Cabau J, Moat N, Colombo A, Latib A (2017) Mechanism and Implications of the Tricuspid Regurgitation. *Circ Cardiovasc Interv.* doi: 10.1161/circinterventions.117.005043.

[22] Brida M, Diller G-P, Gatzoulis MA (2018) Systemic Right Ventricle in Adults with Congenital Heart Disease. *Circulation* 137:508–518.

[23] Bonow RO, Carabello BA, Chatterjee K, et al. (2008) 2008 Focused update incorporated into the ACC/AHA 2006 guidelines for the management of patients with valvular heart disease: a report of the American College of Cardiology/American Heart Association Task Force on Practice Guidelines (Writing Committee to Revise the 1998 Guidelines for the Management of Patients With Valvular Heart Disease): endorsed by the Society of Cardiovascular Anesthesiologists, Society for Cardiovascular Angiography and Interventions, and Society of Thoracic Surgeons. *Circulation* 118:e523-661.

[24] Hung J (2010) The Pathogenesis of Functional Tricuspid Regurgitation. *Semin Thorac Cardiovasc Surg* 22:76–78.

[25] Davlouros PA (2006) The right ventricle in congenital heart disease. *Heart* 92:i27–i38.

[26] Rogers JH, Bolling SF (2009) The tricuspid valve: Current perspective and evolving management of tricuspid regurgitation. *Circulation* 119:2718–2725.

[27] Budts W, Roos-Hesselink J, Rädle-Hurst T, Eicken A, McDonagh TA, Lambrinou E, Crespo-Leiro MG, Walker F, Frogoudaki AA

(2016) Treatment of heart failure in adult congenital heart disease: a position paper of the Working Group of Grown-Up Congenital Heart Disease and the Heart Failure Association of the European Society of Cardiology. *Eur Heart J* 37:1419–1427.

[28] Shah PM (2010) Tricuspid and Pulmonary Valve Disease Evaluation and Management. *Rev Esp Cardiol Engl Ed* 63:1349–1365.

[29] Nikus K, Pérez-Riera AR, Konttila K, Barbosa-Barros R (2018) Electrocardiographic recognition of right ventricular hypertrophy. *J Electrocardiol* 51:46–49.

[30] Nishimura RA, Otto CM, Bonow RO, et al. (2014) 2014 AHA/ACC Guideline for the Management of Patients With Valvular Heart Disease: Executive Summary. *Circulation* 129:2440–2492.

[31] Nishimura RA, Otto CM, Bonow RO, et al. (2017) 2017 AHA/ACC Focused Update of the 2014 AHA/ACC Guideline for the Management of Patients With Valvular Heart Disease: A Report of the American College of Cardiology/American Heart Association Task Force on Clinical Practice Guidelines. *Circulation* 135:e1159–e1195.

[32] Gerche AL, Claessen G, Bruaene AV de, Pattyn N, Cleemput JV, Gewillig M, Bogaert J, Dymarkowski S, Claus P, Heidbuchel H (2013) Cardiac MRI. *Circ Cardiovasc Imaging* 6:329–338.

[33] Baumgartner H, Falk V, Bax JJ, et al. (2017) 2017 ESC/EACTS guidelines for the management of valvular heart disease. *Eur Heart J* 38:2739–2791.

[34] Stout KK, Daniels CJ, Aboulhosn JA, et al. (2019) 2018 AHA/ACC Guideline for the Management of Adults With Congenital Heart Disease: A Report of the American College of Cardiology/American Heart Association Task Force on Clinical Practice Guidelines. *Circulation* 139:e698–e800.

[35] Belluschi I, Forno BD, Lapenna E, Nisi T, Iaci G, Ferrara D, Castiglioni A, Alfieri O, Bonis MD (2018) Surgical Techniques for Tricuspid Valve Disease. *Front Cardiovasc Med.* doi: 10.3389/fcvm. 2018.00118.

[36] De Bonis M, Del Forno B, Nisi T, Lapenna E, Alfieri (2018) Tricuspid valve disease: surgical techniques. In: *Pract. Man. Tricuspid Valve Dis.,* 1st ed. Springer, pp 329–52.

[37] Ross FJ, Latham GJ, Richards M, Geiduschek J, Thompson D, Joffe D (2015) Perioperative and Anesthetic Considerations in Ebstein's Anomaly. *Semin Cardiothorac Vasc Anesth* 20:82–92.

[38] Lange R, Burri M (2017) Surgical Treatment of Ebstein's Anomaly. *Thorac Cardiovasc Surg* 65:639–648.

[39] Said SM, Dearani JA, Burkhart HM, Connolly HM, Eidem B, Stensrud PE, Schaff HV (2014) Management of tricuspid regurgitation in congenital heart disease: Is survival better with valve repair? *J Thorac Cardiovasc Surg* 147:412–419.

[40] Paranon S, Acar P (2008) Ebstein's anomaly of the tricuspid valve: from fetus to adult. *Heart* 94:237–243.

[41] Dearani JA, Mora BN, Nelson TJ, Haile DT, O'Leary PW (2015) Ebstein anomaly review: what's now, what's next? *Expert Rev Cardiovasc Ther* 13:1101–1109.

[42] De León LE, Mery CM, Verm RA, et al. (2017) Mid-Term Outcomes in Patients with Congenitally Corrected Transposition of the Great Arteries: A Single Center Experience. *J Am Coll Surg* 224:707–715.

In: The Rediscovered Tricuspid Valve
Editor: Giacomo Bianchi
ISBN: 978-1-53616-098-7

Chapter 9

NEOPLASTIC DISORDERS INVOLVING THE RIGHT HEART AND THE TRICUSPID VALVE

Angela Pucci*[*], *MD, PhD
Histopathology Department, Pisa University Hospital, Pisa, Italy

ABSTRACT

Primary cardiac tumors are rare whereas metastatic tumors are more frequent. Right heart tumors include a wide range of either primary and secondary (metastatic) neoplasias. The most common primary right heart tumors are biologically benign, but they may manifest with severe hemodynamic and/or arrhythmic symptoms or even sudden death. Most of them are represented by cardiac myxoma (i.e., the most common primary cardiac tumor, mainly affecting the left atrium), by hemangioma (typically affecting the right heart chambers) and by papillary fibroelastoma (usually developing on cardiac valves, first of all the aortic valve). Right-sided primary malignant tumors are mainly constituted by sarcomas and lymphomas. Secondary (metastatic) tumors are mainly represented by carcinomas (firstly lung and breast carcinoma) and sarcomas, but also lymphomas or mesothelioma originating in adjacent structures such as lung, mediastinum or pleura may involve the right heart

[*] Corresponding Author's E-mail: a.pucci@ao-pisa.toscana.it.

structures. The imaging techniques allow diagnosis of most benign and malignant (primary or secondary) cardiac tumors, such as of tumor-like cardiac masses or pseudo-tumors, but the differential diagnosis relies on histology that still represents the gold standard; it is required for definite diagnosis, prognosis and therapeutic management of patients.

Keywords: tricuspid valve, right heart, tumors

Introduction

The heart may be involved by primary or metastatic tumors [1–10]. Primary cardiac tumors are much rarer than metastatic tumors, with a prevalence at autopsy of 0.001-0.03% and of 1.5-2.1%, respectively [11]. About 75% of primary cardiac tumors are biologically benign, surgically resectable and most of them (75% of benign primary cardiac tumors) are constituted by cardiac myxomas [12]. Nevertheless, also benign tumors may have a clinically malignant behavior because of embolism, life-threatening arrhythmias, atrioventricular block, pericardial effusion or tamponade, valvular regurgitation or obstruction, and even sudden death, depending upon their size, site and growth pattern [13–16].

Because symptoms are non-specific and often mimicking other cardiac diseases, their diagnosis may represent a clinical challenge. The improvement of cardiac imaging techniques and the clinical use of echocardiography, together with surgical procedures achievements, including mini-invasive cardiac surgery for resection of cardiac masses [17] have dramatically changed the clinical history of cardiac tumors. Before the 1980s, they represented fatal or incidental post-mortem findings, nowadays most cardiac tumors are diagnosed in vivo and surgery is curative in about 90% of cases [18–23].

Histology concurs to in vivo differential diagnosis, then to prognostic and therapeutic management of cardiac tumors [24, 25]. Although most cardiac masses can be reliably diagnosed by echocardiography and further investigated by other imaging techniques including computed tomography and magnetic resonance, histology is still considered the gold standard for the differential diagnosis that is mandatory in cases requiring exclusion or definite histotype diagnosis of a malignant primary or metastatic tumor. In the last few years, also endomyocardial biopsy and very recently vacuum aspiration techniques in selected cases (such as caval vein embolism from a renal cell carcinoma; personal experience) may be valuable tools for the differential diagnosis in unresectable tumors by means of histology and ancillary immunohistochemical or molecular techniques that may be crucial [26].

Primary cardiac tumors are world-wide classified according to the World Health Organization guidelines. The most frequent primary cardiac tumors are the biologically benign cardiac myxomas, followed by papillary fibroelastomas, mainly involving the left atrium and the cardiac valves, respectively [2, 7, 8]. Many other benign tumors may affect the heart. As to malignant tumors, the most frequent primary malignant tumors of the heart are represented by sarcomas, followed by lymphomas [5, 6]. Cardiac sarcomas arise from the right side of the heart in 25% of reported cases, whereas myxomas arise from right-sided cardiac structures in only 15% of cases. Then, an intracavitary tumor involving the right heart and/or obstructing the right ventricular outflow tract is more likely to be malignant than left-sided tumor [27]. We herein focus on the most clinically significant tumors with a particular focus on neoplasisas that can involve or affect the valve.

Primary Right Heart Tumors

Cardiac Myxoma

Cardiac myxoma represents the most common primary cardiac tumor. It is more frequent in the inter-atrial septum of the left atrium (about 75% of cases), followed by the right atrium (15-29%), then by ventricles and other cardiac structures [12, 28–32]. Mean age at presentation is 50 years with a slight female preponderance (F/M ratio of 1.8/1), but it has been described at any (including neonatal) age. They are usually solitary tumors (90% of cases), rarely multiple and/or familial as part of the Carney Complex that is an autosomal dominant syndrome (with PRKAR1A gene mutations in chromosome 2) associated with spotty skin pigmentation, blue nevus, endocrinopathy, endocrine and non-endocrine tumors including cardiac, cutaneous and breast myxomas [29, 30]. This intra-cardiac tumor has a highly variable size, mean maximum diameter ranging between 5 and 7 cm, gross features corresponding to a smooth, oval and lobulated or villous, friable and gelatinous-like mass. Its diagnosis is usually performed by echocardiography and its more frequent presenting symptoms are embolic phenomena (pulmonary embolism in the right-sided tumors), followed by valve stenosis, syncope and even sudden death, although they may be asymptomatic and represent incidental findings [33–37].

Histology show an amorphous mucopolysaccharide-rich matrix (conferring the typical myxoid aspect) with numerous thin blood vessels and the characteristic lepidic cells, i.e., polygonal cells that are embedded within the myxoid stroma as scattered cells, small nests or perivascular cuff (Figure 1). By immunohistochemistry, these cells show strong immunoreactivity for S100 and Calretinin; their identification is a diagnostic clue, also for differential diagnosis from malignant myxoid sarcomas (later described).

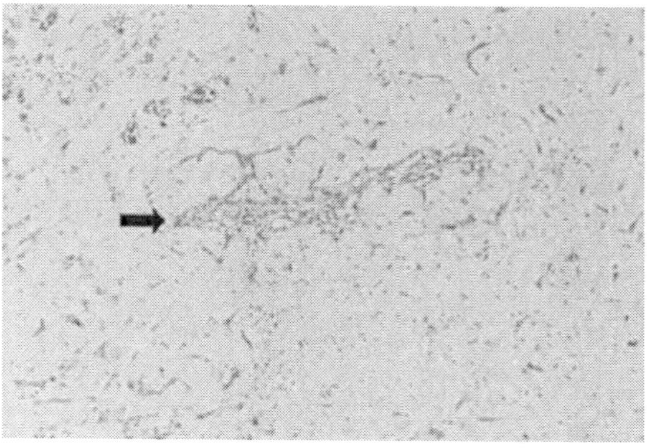

Figure 1. Right atrial myxoma. In the amorphous mucopolysaccharide-rich matrix (conferring the typical myxoid aspect) the characteristic lepidic cells (arrow) are embedded within the myxoid stroma as a perivascular cuff (Haematoxylin and Eosin staining; original magnification: 4x.

Cardiac myxomas may show extensive calcification (lithomyxoma), pseudo-lymphomatous proliferations [38] or glandular components [39] mimicking a malignant primary or metastatic tumor; in such cases identification of the lepidic component may be necessary for the definite differential diagnosis. Molecular studies and confocal microscopy have contributed to establish their true neoplastic nature and their differentiation pattern, their cell of origin being very likely represented by mesenchymal multipotent cells [25, 40].

TRICUSPID VALVE:
BENIGN TUMORS AND PSEUDO-TUMORS

Primary cardiac valve tumors are extremely rare, their reported incidence representing less than 10% of all primary cardiac tumors [41–43]. Anyhow, they are gradually becoming less rare because of diagnostic technologies progress. They usually have a smaller size, greater mobility, and more tendency to embolize than the intramural tumors. Fibroelastoma is the most common valvular tumor, followed by myxoma [44]. Cardiac valve may also harbor non-neoplastic lesions that mimic tumors, the so-called pseudo-tumors that usually affect elder patients.

Cardiac valve tumors and pseudo-tumors usually have a small size and a little influence on related leaflet function, but prompt surgical resection is mandatory for prevention of embolic events, accounting for approximately 0.34% of adult cardiac operations.

Papillary Fibroelastoma

Most tricuspid valve tumors are papillary fibroelastomas that constitute the second cause of benign cardiac tumors [44–47]. Their true incidence is unknown. The tricuspid valve is less commonly affected than the other cardiac valvular structures; the aortic valve represents the most frequent site (52%), followed by the mitral valve (16%), then by the pulmonary and by the tricuspid valve. Papillary fibroelastoma of the tricuspid valve is usually <1 cm maximum diameter and show a short stalk with high mobility that may explain the relatively frequent embolic events. It can be detected by echocardiography and histology is usually required for differential diagnosis from other tumors or pseudo-tumors, first thrombus.

At gross examination, it is a white-gray, soft mass, sometimes with brownish areas due to the frequent occurrence of superimposed thrombus. Papillary fibroelastomas display multiple papillary fronds resulting in a sea-anemone feature by water immersion. At microscopic level, each frond is constituted by an endothelial lining (as demonstrated by CD31 or CD34 positive immunostaining) covering a fibromyxoid core with a prominent elastic fiber component as demonstrated by histochemical Weigert or elastic van Gieson staining (Figure 2).

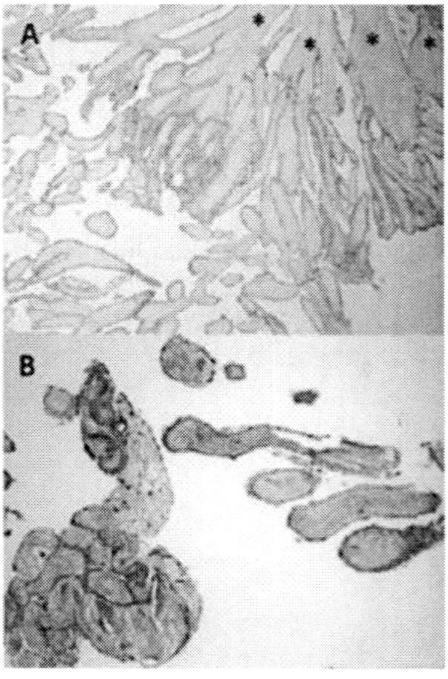

Figure 2. Tricuspid valve papillaruy fibroelastoma. Multiple papillary fronds (*) constituted by an endothelial lining covering a fibromyxoid core with a prominent elastic fiber component as demonstrated by histochemical Weigert staining (a: Haematoxylin and Eosin staining, original magnification 4x; b: Weigert staining, original magnification 4x).

Tricuspid Valve Myxomas

These tumors are exceedingly rare accounting for 8.8% of cardiac myxomas [41, 42]. They are macroscopically gelatinous, lobulated tumors, often solitary with a short stalk, and are diagnosed by echocardiography [14, 19, 24]. Tricuspid valve myxoma show the same histologic features as right atrial myxomas [48] (see following section). Surgical excision is recommended for embolization risk.

Tricuspid Valve Lipoma and Lipomatous Hamartoma

Although most reported cases involve aortic or mitral valve [49], the tricuspid valve may be a site of large lipomas involving the inter-atrial septum and/or other right cardiac structures (i.e., ventricular myocardium) [50]. They may be represented by an exophytic, well-delimited lesion (lipoma) or by an infiltrating lipomatous proliferation (better defined as lipomatous hamartoma), displacing the fibrous core of the tricuspid valve. Histologic features are similar to lipomas/lipomatous proliferations in other cardiac structures, i.e., they are constituted by lobules of mature adipocytes with thin fibrous septa and no cell atypia or expression of MDM2.

Tricuspid Valve Hemangioma

This tumor has been exceptionally reported in the Tricuspid Valve [51–55]. Either capillary and cavernous hemangiomas have been shown, in both adulthood and neonatal age. The size of the tricuspid valve hemangiomas varies from 0.1 to 3 cm; they are usually single lesions with variable mode of presentation, from asymptomatic ones to cases with dyspnea, regurgitation and even severe cardio-respiratory distress. They have been reported after successful surgical removal, but also in a case of sudden infant death syndrome associated with hypoplastic left ventricle syndrome.

Tricuspid Valve Pseudotumors

Tricuspid valve pseudotumors are non-neoplastic masses including organized thrombus, valvular calcifications and the calcified amorphous tumor (CAT), valvular abscesses; they show symptoms and morphological features that look similar to the valvular tumors in a usually elder patients' group [8].

Cardiac thrombi are more common than tumors; they require timely diagnosis and treatment. Valvular thrombus on the tricuspid valve is usually mobile and small (about 1 cm diameter), mainly sessile without a stalk, but rarely valvular thrombi may have a pedicle and be larger than 2 cm. Equivocal findings by echocardiography might be ascertained by magnetic resonance imaging.

The *Calcified Amorphous Tumor* (CAT) is a non-neoplastic, intracavitary lesion, frequently associated with valve disease (31%), concomitant mitral annulus calcifications (14%) or coronary artery disease (12%), but also with end-stage renal disease (21%) and diabetes (14%) [56]. By echocardiography, CAT is usually shown as a calcified endocavitary mass of variable size (from small punctate lesions to very large masses) in any cardiac chamber, valve or valvular annulus. By imaging, CAT can be mistaken for osteosarcoma, calcified myxoma (lithomyxoma) or endocarditic vegetations. For the definite diagnosis, histology is required [57]. The histopathologic investigations show nodular calcium deposits surrounded by an amorphous hyalinized material, plus variable plasma cells and lymphocytic infiltrates in a fibrous stroma without cell atypia (Figure 3).

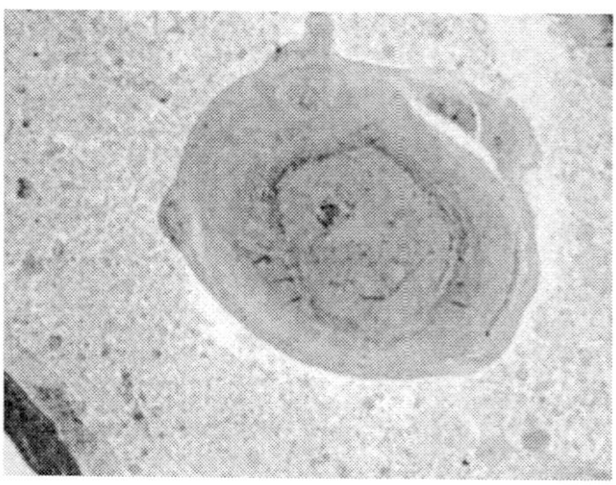

Figure 3. Tricuspid valve calciphied amorphous tumor (CAT). Nodular calcium deposits surrounded by an amorphous hyalinized material (Haematoxylin and Eosin staining; original magnification: 4x).

Valvular calcifications, CAT and abscesses are usually associated with severe valve dysfunction; in most cases they are easily distinguished from valvular tumors by echocardiography. However, in atypical cases, these lesions such as CAT might be tumor-like and make diagnoses difficult before surgery [58]. Such cases may require histology for differential diagnosis.

Malignant Right Heart and Tricuspid Valve Tumors

The tricuspid valve can be involved by malignant tumors such as sarcomas and lymphomas, variously spreading to the right heart chambers [2, 59–61].

Sarcomas

Cardiac sarcoma represents the most frequent primary malignant tumor of the heart, so far [5]. Angiosarcoma is the most common primary cardiac sarcoma in adults and most cases occur in the right atrium [62]. Depending on the site involved, sarcomas can present with different symptoms, including dyspnea, cough, chest discomfort, orthopnea or syncope, heart failure, pericardial effusion with/without tamponade, arrhythmias, valvular abnormalities or obstructive symptoms. In right-sided cardiac sarcomas, pulmonary embolism can be the presenting feature. They may present as a broad-based lesion, often infiltrating the myocardium, pericardium or adjacent structures and may involve an entire cardiac chamber. The diagnosis of malignancy is usually established using non-invasive imaging modalities such as echocardiography (TTE or TEE). CT scan and MRI are useful for assessment of tumor characteristics and to investigate presence of metastases, myocardial infiltration, pericardial and great vessel involvement [63]. Definitive diagnosis requires histology to differentiate them from other tumors such as NHL or even benign but infiltrating tumors or pseudo-tumors with different therapeutic management and prognosis. Tissue biopsy for histological diagnosis may be obtained through endomyocardial biopsy, endoscopy, mediastinoscopy or thoracotomy. By means of histology and ancillary techniques, i.e., immunohistochemistry and molecular pathology, the sarcomas are classified according to the WHO.

Angiosarcomas is usually a cauliflower-like, dark red mass protruding into the right atrial cavity, often infiltrating pericardium at diagnosis and causing hemorrhagic pericardial effusion and even tamponade. It may obstruct the tricuspid valve and extend into the right ventricle. Histologically, it may form variously anastomosed vascular channels with atypical endothelial cells, in the more differentiated forms, or (in one third of cases) be poorly differentiated and mainly constituted by spindle cells with endothelial differentiation as demonstrated by immunohistochemistry (immunoreactivity for specific antibodies raised against endothelial cell markers, i.e., CD31, FVIII Rag, CD34) (Figure 4).

Besides angiosarcomas, different sarcomas have been described in the right atrium, either differentiated sarcomas including liposarcoma, synovial sarcoma, leiomyosarcoma, osteosarcoma, and undifferentiated (pleomorphic or spindle cell) sarcomas [10].

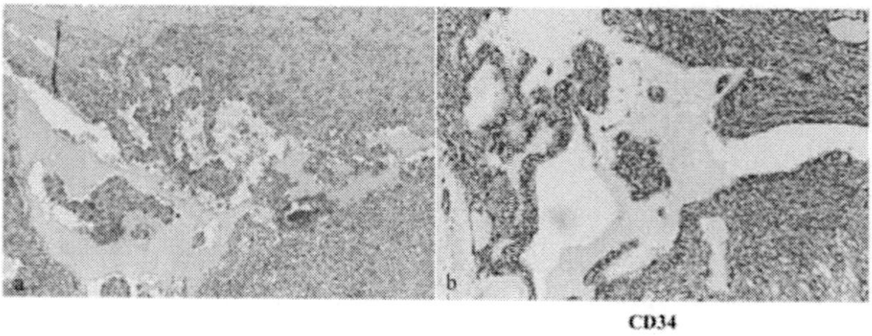

Figure 4. Right atrial angiosarcoma. Variously anastomosed vascular channels with atypical endothelial cells (a); endothelial differentiation is demonstrated by immunohistochemistry, i.e., immunoreactivity for CD31 endothelial cell marker (a: Haematoxylin and Eosin staining; b: Immunoperoxidase staining; original magnification: 4x).

The undifferentiated sarcomas lack a specific histology, no cell lineage differentiation or specific gene mutation being demonstrated by immunohistochemistry or molecular pathology techniques, respectively.

Although the prognosis of sarcomas depends on tumor grading, established according to FNCLCC score system (based on the mitotic activity, necrosis and cellular differentiation), the cardiac sarcomas show an aggressive behavior and still have a poor prognosis with a mean survival of <12 months [64]. Only few anecdotical cases with long (up to 11 years) survival have been reported [65]. The poor prognosis is very likely related to a late diagnosis with impossible radical resection in many cases, whereas tumor subtyping does not apparently affect the overall clinical outcome of primary cardiac sarcomas. Although surgery remains the only treatment, adjuvant therapeutic methods are under investigation.

Lymphoma

Primary cardiac lymphomas account for less than 0.01% of all cardiac tumors and are represented by Non-Hodgkin Lymphomas (NHL) involving exclusively the heart and/or the pericardium [59, 61]. The right atrium represents the most common site of origin of primary cardiac NHLs, although they may involve any cardiac chamber and structure by infiltrating the myocardium and sometimes diffusing into the pericardium. The mean age is 62 years with a wide age range (5-90 years). Onset symptoms are various and non-specific, including shortness of breath, palpitations, chest pain, syncope, arrhythmias, congestive heart failure or pericardial effusion. Almost 80% of cases are represented by diffuse large B-cell NHL that show CD20 positive large lymphocytes with high proliferating (Ki67 or MIB1) index, followed by T-cell (CD^{3+}) NHL and by Burkitt-like NHL (Figure 5).

These tumors are considered highly aggressive, and are treated as their non-cardiac counterparts, by chemotherapy. In recent series, after first-line chemotherapy, a complete response was obtained in 62% of patients, recurrences occurred in 55% of patients, and the aggressiveness of primary cardiac lymphomas has been related also to the possible onset of acute cardiac events [66, 67].

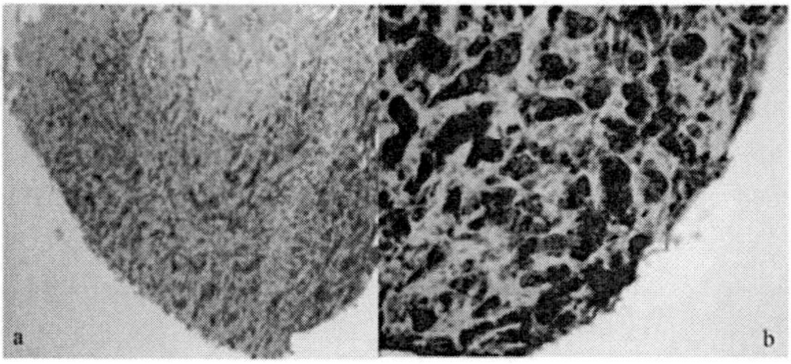

Figure 5. Right atrium, diffuse large B-cell non-Hodgkin lymphoma. Diffuse infiltration of the myocardium by large and atypical B-cell (a) that are positive (b) for CD20 B-cell antigen (a: Haematoxylin and Eosin staining, original magnification 4x; b: Immunoperoxidase staining, original magnification: 10x).

Metastatic Right Heart Tumors

Metastases to the heart and pericardium are much more common than primary cardiac tumors, they usually carry a poor prognosis, but they may go unrecognized without autopsy [11, 68–70].

The malignant neoplasias more frequently metastatizing or extending to the heart (including pericardium) are the lung and breast carcinomas, followed by melanoma and lymphoma. The incidence of malignant pericardial involvement has been reported in the Literature ranging between 0.15%–21% of all patients with an underlying malignancy. It is estimated that of all patients with malignant cardiac involvement, about 85% have pericardial involvement.

Cardiac metastases may have retrograde lymphatic extension, hematogenous spread, direct contiguous or transvenous extension. In 30% patients with cardiac metastases, impaired cardiac function is related to neoplastic pericardial effusion.

The clinical presentation includes shortness of breath, cough, anterior thoracic pain, pleuritic chest pain or peripheral edema. On the other hand, in a patient with known malignancy the differential diagnosis of pericardial effusion includes malignant pericardial effusion, radiation-induced pericarditis, drug-induced pericarditis, and idiopathic pericarditis. Prognosis is usually poor with survival after diagnosis ranging from six weeks to 15 months.

Endocardial metastases show a predilection for the right chambers of the heart (right atrium and ventricle) and the most frequent primitive neoplasia are renal cell carcinoma, hepatocellular carcinoma and uterine tumors (via inferior caval vein) or thyroid tumors (via superior caval vein). Valve metastases are very rare (likely because of continuous cuspid motion and absence of vessels) or show a neoplastic thrombotic endocarditis.

Myocardial metastases do not apparently show a preferential site of involvement. According to some Authors, the right ventricle is particularly affected because of lower pressure and systolic function, favoring metastatic lodging [70]. Tipically, NHLs may secondarily involve the atrial and ventricular walls.

Epicardial metastases usually look like nodular or diffuse infiltration, they occur secondarily to pericardial metastases (see the following section), via lymphatic pathway (particularly evident in areas with impaired lymphatic drainage secondary to cardiac dysfunction) or bloodstream.

Pericardial metastases may show a focal, diffuse or massive involvement of the pericardium. Besides various tumors (metastatic carcinomas and sarcomas via bloodstream or lymphatic pathway, pleural mesothelioma by direct extension) also Hodgkin Lymphoma has been shown to involve the pericardium (more than myocardium that is a site of NHLs). Metastatic carcinomas and adenocarcinomas may require differential diagnosis from epithelioid mesothelioma; such diagnosis usually relies on histological investigations, including immunohistochemistry.

Conclusion

The right heart can be a site of primary or secondary neoplasia, a few tumors (including malignant sarcomas) showing right-sided cardiac chambers and/or valve structures to represent a preferential site. The differential diagnosis of an intracardiac mass includes thrombus, benign or malignant tumors, and infectious or inflammatory masses. Non-invasive imaging tests give important diagnostic clues, but tissue biopsy and histology (including ancillary techniques) are necessary for the differential diagnosis. A multi-disciplinary approach is paramount in managing cardiac masses.

References

[1] Roberts WC (1997) Primary and Secondary Neoplasms of the Heart. *Am J Cardiol* 80:671–682.

[2] McAllister HA, Hall RJ, Cooley DA (1999) Tumors of the heart and pericardium. *Curr Probl Cardiol* 24:59–116.

[3] Neragi-Miandoab S, Kim J, Vlahakes GJ (2007) Malignant Tumours of the Heart: A Review of Tumour Type, Diagnosis and Therapy. *Clin Oncol* 19:748–756.

[4] Al-Mamgani A, Baartman L, Baaijens M, Pree I de, Incrocci L, Levendag PC (2008) Cardiac metastases. *Int J Clin Oncol* 13:369–372.

[5] Burke A (2008) Primary malignant cardiac tumors. *Semin Diagn Pathol* 25:39–46.

[6] Burke A, Jeudy J, Virmani R (2008) Cardiac tumours: an update. *Heart* 94:117–123.

[7] Simpson L, Kumar SK, Okuno SH, Schaff HV, Porrata LF, Buckner JC, Moynihan TJ (2008) Malignant primary cardiac tumors. *Cancer* 112:2440–2446

[8] Bruce CJ (2010) Cardiac tumours: diagnosis and management. *Heart* 97:151–160.

[9] Burnside N, MacGowan SW (2012) Malignant primary cardiac tumours. *Interact Cardiovasc Thorac Surg* 15:1004–1006.

[10] Travis WD, Brambilla E, Burke AP, Marx A, Nicholson AG (2015) Introduction to The 2015 World Health Organization Classification of Tumors of the Lung, Pleura, Thymus, and Heart. *J Thorac Oncol* 10:1240–1242.

[11] Reynen K (1996) Frequency of primary tumors of the heart. *Am J Cardiol* 77:107.

[12] Reynen K (1995) Cardiac myxomas. *N Engl J Med* 333:1610–1617.

[13] Cina SJ, Smialek JE, Burke AP, Virmani R, Hutchins GM (1996) Primary Cardiac Tumors Causing Sudden Death: A Review of the Literature. *Am J Forensic Med Pathol* 17:271–281.

[14] Pucci A, Gagliardotto P, Zanini C, Pansini S, di Summa M, Mollo F (2000) Histopathologic and clinical characterization of cardiac myxoma: review of 53 cases from a single institution. *Am Heart J* 140:134–138.

[15] Pucci A, Botta G, Sina N, et al., (2013) Life-Threatening Tumors of the Heart in Fetal and Postnatal Age. *J Pediatr* 162:964–969.e1.

[16] ElBardissi AW, Dearani JA, Daly RC, Mullany CJ, Orszulak TA, Puga FJ, Schaff HV (2009) Embolic Potential of Cardiac Tumors and Outcome After Resection. *Stroke* 40:156–162.

[17] Bianchi G, Margaryan R, Kallushi E, Cerillo AG, Farneti PA, Pucci A, Solinas M (2019) Outcomes of Video-assisted Minimally Invasive Cardiac Myxoma Resection. *Heart Lung Circ* 28:327–333.

[18] Sarjeant JM, Butany J, Cusimano RJ (2003) Cancer of the Heart. *Am J Cardiovasc Drugs* 3:407–421.

[19] Kirkpatrick JN, Wong T, Bednarz JE, Spencer KT, Sugeng L, Ward RP, DeCara JM, Weinert L, Krausz T, Lang RM (2004) Differential diagnosis of cardiac masses using contrast echocardiographic perfusion imaging. *J Am Coll Cardiol* 43:1412–1419.

[20] Elbardissi AW, Dearani JA, Daly RC, Mullany CJ, Orszulak TA, Puga FJ, Schaff HV (2008) Survival after resection of primary cardiac tumors: a 48-year experience. *Circulation* 118:S7-15.

[21] Mansencal N, Revault-d'Allonnes L, Pelage JP, Farcot JC, Lacombe P, Dubourg O (2009) Usefulness of contrast echocardiography for assessment of intracardiac masses. *Arch Cardiovasc Dis* 102:177–183.

[22] Patel R, Lim RP, Saric M, Nayar A, Babb J, Ettel M, Axel L, Srichai MB (2016) Diagnostic Performance of Cardiac Magnetic Resonance Imaging and Echocardiography in Evaluation of Cardiac and Paracardiac Masses. *Am J Cardiol* 117:135–140.

[23] Zaragoza-Macias E, Zaidi AN, Dendukuri N, Marelli A (2019) Medical Therapy for Systemic Right Ventricles: A Systematic Review (Part 1) for the 2018 AHA/ACC Guideline for the Management of Adults with Congenital Heart Disease. *J Am Coll Cardiol* 73:1564–1578.

[24] Meng Q, Lai H, Lima J, Tong W, Qian Y, Lai S (2002) Echocardiographic and pathologic characteristics of primary cardiac tumors: a study of 149 cases. *Int J Cardiol* 84:69–75.

[25] Pucci A, Mattioli C, Matteucci M, et al., (2018) Cell differentiation in cardiac myxomas: confocal microscopy and gene expression analysis after laser capture microdissection. *Heart Vessels* 33:1403–1410.

[26] Leone O, Veinot JP, Angelini A, et al., (2012) 2011 Consensus statement on endomyocardial biopsy from the Association for European Cardiovascular Pathology and the Society for Cardiovascular Pathology. *Cardiovasc Pathol* 21:245–274.

[27] Gopal AS, Arora NS, Messineo FC (2000) Right Ventricular Myxoma. *N Engl J Med* 342:295–295.

[28] St John Sutton MG, Mercier LA, Giuliani ER, Lie JT (1980) Atrial myxomas: a review of clinical experience in 40 patients. *Mayo Clin Proc Mayo Clin* 55:371–376.

[29] Carney JA, Gordon H, Carpenter PC, Shenoy BV, Go VL (1985) The complex of myxomas, spotty pigmentation, and endocrine overactivity. *Medicine* (Baltimore) 64:270–283.

[30] Vidaillet HJ, Seward JB, Fyke FE, Su WP, Tajik AJ (1987) "Syndrome myxoma": a subset of patients with cardiac myxoma associated with pigmented skin lesions and peripheral and endocrine neoplasms. *Heart* 57:247–255.

[31] Pinede L, Duhaut P, Loire R (2001) Clinical presentation of left atrial cardiac myxoma. A series of 112 consecutive cases. *Medicine* (Baltimore) 80:159–172.

[32] Bartoloni G, Pucci A (2012) Cardiac Myxoma. In: *Card. Tumor Pathol.* Humana Press, pp 31–44.

[33] Bhan A, Mehrotra R, Choudhary SK, Sharma R, Prabhakar D, Airan B, Kumar AS, Venugopal P (1998) Surgical experience with intracardiac myxomas: long-term follow-up. *Ann Thorac Surg* 66:810–813.

[34] Keeling I (2002) Cardiac myxomas: 24 years of experience in 49 patients. *Eur J Cardiothorac Surg* 22:971–977.

[35] Lee VH, Connolly HM, Brown RD (2007) Central Nervous System Manifestations of Cardiac Myxoma. *Arch Neurol* 64:1115.

[36] D'Alfonso A, Catania S, Pierri MD, Matteucci SL, Rescigno G, Münch C, Staine J, Iacobone G, Piccoli GP (2008) Atrial myxoma: a 25-year single-institutional follow-up study. *J Cardiovasc Med* 9:178–181.

[37] Shah IK, Dearani JA, Daly RC, Suri RM, Park SJ, Joyce LD, Li Z, Schaff HV (2015) Cardiac Myxomas: A 50-Year Experience With Resection and Analysis of Risk Factors for Recurrence. *Ann Thorac* Surg 100:495–500.

[38] Bartoloni G, Pucci A, Giorlandino A, Berretta M, Mignosa C, Italia F, Carbone A, Canzonieri V (2013) Incidental Epstein–Barr virus associated atypical lymphoid proliferation arising in a left atrial myxoma: a case of long survival without any postsurgical treatment and review of the literature. *Cardiovasc Pathol* 22:e5–e10.

[39] Pucci A, Bartoloni G, Tessitore E, Carney JA, Papotti M (2003) Cytokeratin profile and neuroendocrine cells in the glandular component of cardiac myxoma. *Virchows Arch* 443:618–624.

[40] Orlandi A, Ciucci A, Ferlosio A, Pellegrino A, Chiariello L, Spagnoli LG (2005) Increased Expression and Activity of Matrix Metalloproteinases Characterize Embolic Cardiac Myxomas. *Am J Pathol* 166:1619–1628.

[41] Edwards FH, Hale D, Cohen A, Thompson L, Pezzella AT, Virmani R (1991) Primary cardiac valve tumors. *Ann Thorac Surg* 52:1127–1131.

[42] Basso C (2003) Primary cardiac valve tumours. *Heart* 89:1259–1260.

[43] Wang Y, Wang X, Xiao Y (2016) Surgical treatment of primary cardiac valve tumor: early and late results in eight patients. *J Cardiothorac Surg.* doi: 10.1186/s13019-016-0406-2.

[44] Tamin SS, Maleszewski JJ, Scott CG, Khan SK, Edwards WD, Bruce CJ, Oh JK, Pellikka PA, Klarich KW (2015) Prognostic and Bioepidemiologic Implications of Papillary Fibroelastomas. *J Am Coll Cardiol* 65:2420–2429.

[45] Klarich KW, Enriquez-Sarano M, Gura GM, Edwards WD, Tajik AJ, Seward JB (1997) Papillary Fibroelastoma: Echocardiographic Characteristics for Diagnosis and Pathologic Correlation. *J Am Coll Cardiol* 30:784–790.

[46] Sun JP, Asher CR, Yang XS, Cheng GG, Scalia GM, Massed AG, Griffin BP, Ratliff NB, Stewart WJ, Thomas JD (2001) Clinical and Echocardiographic Characteristics of Papillary Fibroelastomas. *Circulation* 103:2687–2693.

[47] Gowda RM, Khan IA, Nair CK, Mehta NJ, Vasavada BC, Sacchi TJ (2003) Cardiac papillary fibroelastoma: a comprehensive analysis of 725 cases. *Am Heart J* 146:404–410.

[48] Sabzi F, Ghasemi F, Asadmobini A (2016) A Tricuspid Valve Mass Attached to Papillary Muscle. *Ethiop J Health Sci* 26:293.

[49] Martino AD, Blasi S, Lorenzini D, Fornaro M, Basolo F, Bortolotti U, Pucci A (2016) Lipomatous hamartoma-like lesion of a bicuspid

aortic valve: an incidental surgical finding. *Cardiovasc Pathol* 25:500–502.

[50] Fang L, He L, Chen Y, Xie M, Wang J (2016) Infiltrating Lipoma of the Right Ventricle Involving the Interventricular Septum and Tricuspid Valve. *Medicine* (Baltimore) 95:e2561.

[51] Lapenna E, Bonis MD, Torracca L, Canna GL, Dell'Antonio G, Alfieri O (2003) Cavernous hemangioma of the tricuspid valve: minimally invasive surgical resection. *Ann Thorac Surg* 76:2097–2099.

[52] Ray R, Rishi A, Venugopal P, Chopra P (2004) Hemangioma of the tricuspid valve. *Cardiovasc Patho*l 13:120–122.

[53] Cannata A, Russo CF, Merlanti B, Pedrotti P, Moreo A, Botta L, Martinelli L (2010) Cavernous Hemangioma Replacing the Septal Leaflet of the Tricuspid Valve. *J Card Surg* 25:524–527.

[54] Floria M, Guedes A, Buche M, Deperon R, Marchandise B (2011) A rare primary cardiac tumour: cavernous hemangioma of the tricuspid valve. *Eur Heart J - Cardiovasc Imaging* 12:477–477.

[55] Gupta B, Ghosh S, Kujur M, Khetan K, Kumar T (2016) Tricuspid valve hemangioma associated with hypoplastic left heart syndrome presenting as sudden infant death syndrome. *Turk J Pathol.* doi: 10.5146/tjpath.2015.01362.

[56] Reynolds C, Tazelaar HD, Edwards WD (1997) Calcified amorphous tumor of the heart (cardiac CAT). *Hum Pathol* 28:601–606.

[57] Hemptinne Q de, Cannière D de, Vandenbossche JL, Unger P (2015) Cardiac calcified amorphous tumor: A systematic review of the literature. *IJC Heart Vasc* 7:1–5.

[58] Yuan S-M, Jing H, Lavee J (2009) Tumors and tumor-like lesions of the heart valves. *Rare Tumors* 1:105–109.

[59] Petersen CD, Robinson WA, Kurnick JE (1976) Involvement of the heart and pericardium in the malignant lymphomas. *Am J Med Sci* 272:161–165.

[60] Truong PT, Jones SO, Martens B, Alexander C, Paquette M, Joe H, Hart J, Allan SJ (2009) Treatment and Outcomes in Adult Patients

with Primary Cardiac Sarcoma: The British Columbia Cancer Agency Experience. *Ann Surg Oncol* 16:3358–3365.

[61] Miguel CE, Bestetti RB (2011) Primary cardiac lymphoma. *Int J Cardiol* 149:358–363.

[62] Butany J, Yu W (2000) Cardiac angiosarcoma: two cases and a review of the literature. *Can J Cardiol* 16:197–205.

[63] Kupsky DF, Newman DB, Kumar G, Maleszewski JJ, Edwards WD, Klarich KW (2015) Echocardiographic Features of Cardiac Angiosarcomas: The Mayo Clinic Experience (1976-2013). *Echocardiography* 33:186–192.

[64] Bakaeen FG, Jaroszewski DE, Rice DC, Walsh GL, Vaporciyan AA, Swisher SS, Benjamin R, Blackmon S, Reardon MJ (2009) Outcomes after surgical resection of cardiac sarcoma in the multimodality treatment era. *J Thorac Cardiovasc Surg* 137:1454–1460.

[65] Modi A, Lipnevicius A, Moorjani N, Haw M (2009) Prolonged survival with left atrial spindle cell sarcoma. *Interact Cardiovasc Thorac Surg* 8:703–704.

[66] Cikirikcioglu M, Keil V, Cherian S, Theologou T, Merlani P, Muller H, Licker MJ, Kalangos A (2011) Primary Cardiac Lymphoma Causing Right Atrial Occlusion. *Thorac Cardiovasc Surg* 59:173–175.

[67] Carras S, Berger F, Chalabreysse L, Callet-Bauchut E, Cordier J-F, Salles G, Girard N (2016) Primary cardiac lymphoma: diagnosis, treatment and outcome in a modern series. *Hematol Oncol* 35:510–519.

[68] Bortolotti U, Caiabró F, Loy M, Fasoli G, Altavilla G, Marchese D (1992) Giant intrapericardial solitary fibrous tumor. *Ann Thorac Surg* 54:1219–1220.

[69] Reynen K, Köckeritz U, Strasser RH (2004) Metastases to the heart. *Ann Oncol Off J Eur Soc Med Oncol* 15:375–381.

[70] Bussani R, De-Giorgio F, Abbate A, Silvestri F (2007) Cardiac metastases. *J Clin Pathol* 60:27–34.

In: The Rediscovered Tricuspid Valve ISBN: 978-1-53616-098-7
Editor: Giacomo Bianchi

Chapter 10

PHARMACOLOGICAL TREATMENT OF TRICUSPID REGURGITATION

Alberto Aimo*[*]*, MD, Luigi Francesco Saccaro, MD, Valentina Galfo, MD, Lucio Teresi, MD and Michele Emdin, MD, PhD

Institute of Life Sciences, Scuola Superiore Sant'Anna, Pisa, Italy

ABSTRACT

When not caused by acute conditions, tricuspid regurgitation (TR) is generally characterized by long asymptomatic phases accompanied by increase in+ hemodynamic severity. Severe TR leads to right ventricular (RV) pressure and volume overload culminating in RV failure, which is a strong predictor of adverse outcome. First-line treatment of severe TR is valve repair or replacement. No rigorous evidence supports pharmacological therapy for TR, although drug therapies may be appropriate in acute TR, or as a bridge to intervention in decompensated patients. While diuretics are obviously mandatory for patients with signs of RV failure, the only other recommended approach is the reduction of elevated pulmonary artery pressures and/or pulmonary vascular

[*] Corresponding Author's E-mail: albertoaimo@libero.it.

resistances in severe functional TR. The therapeutic goals of medical treatment for TR should be treating dysfunctional ventricle(s), reducing pulmonary and/or peripheral congestion while avoiding RV underfilling, and relieving pulmonary hypertension: strategies to achieve these goals allow symptom control and patient stabilization, but are not disease-modifying therapies, with the possible exception of neurohormonal antagonists. For this reason, medical treatment should not delay surgery to avoid the development of irreversible RV dysfunction. When patients are not candidates to surgery, percutaneous treatment of TR should be preferred over medical therapy alone.

Keywords: tricuspid valve, medical treatment, pharmacology

INTRODUCTION

Tricuspid regurgitation (TR) is the most common lesion of the tricuspid valve, occurring in 65-85% of the general population [1]. TR is classified as primary (organic) or secondary (functional). Primary TR is caused by structural abnormalities of the TV, while secondary TR derives from annular dilatation and/or increased right ventricular (RV) eccentricity. Organic or primary TR is due to structural damage of the valvular apparatus. It may be caused by acquired (such as infective endocarditis, carcinoid infiltration, rheumatic heart valve disease, trauma), iatrogenic (such as central catheters, endocardial device leads), or congenital (e.g., TV dysplasia, Ebstein's anomaly) conditions [2, 3]. Among the causes of secondary TR there are conditions of right heart dysfunction (such as longstanding atrial fibrillation, RV ischemia, sarcoidosis, or arrhythmogenic RV cardiomyopathy), and pulmonary hypertension (because of acute pulmonary embolism, primary disorders of the lungs, left ventricle - LV, mitral or aortic valves) [4, 5].

TR severity is proportional to tricuspid annular dilatation and RV eccentricity [6, 7], but also RV contractility and loading conditions (both preload and afterload) [8]. TR also exposes the right atrium to higher volumes and pressures, promoting the onset of atrial fibrillation, which in turn may promote annular dilatation. Additionally, moderate-to-severe TR causes a pressure and volume overload, which further depresses RV function, thus creating a vicious cycle. Indeed, the traditional teaching that functional TR resolves upon correction of the underlying disease has proven to be incorrect [9]. On the contrary, TR is a progressive disease, when left untreated [10]. Worsening of TR is less likely in patients with mild TR, no prominent leaflet tethering, annular dilatation, and on sinus rhythm [1, 11]. Although it might be well tolerated for years, there is a gradual decrease in survival free from cardiac events with increasing TR severity [12, 13], while TR jet area is an independent determinant of mortality in patients with isolated TR [14].

Patients with moderate-to-severe TR may develop signs and symptoms of RV failure, with peripheral edema, ascites, jugular vein congestion, hepatic congestion, dyspnea, fatigue, and reduced tolerance to exercise [15]. At rest, pulmonary capillary wedge pressure (PCWP) and right atrial pressure are higher than in healthy controls, whereas pulmonary blood flow is lower. During exercise, patients with TR display insufficient LV diastolic filling, lower peak oxygen consumption, a smaller increase in pulmonary blood flow, and increased PCWP [16].

Guideline Recommendations and Goals of Pharmacological Treatment

TR treatment is mainly surgical, and valve repair is generally preferable to valve substitution. Surgical correction should be performed before irreversible RV dysfunction develops [17]. The indications for surgery are discussed in detail in dedicated chapters, and recommendations from European Society of Cardiology (ESC) and American Heart Association (AHA).

While there is a general agreement that pharmacological therapy should not delay surgery [18], ESC Guidelines do not provide any specific recommendation on drug treatment [17]. However, AHA Guidelines include two C level of evidence recommendations for diuretic therapy in patients with severe TR and signs of right-sided HF (class IIa), and drugs to reduce elevated pulmonary artery pressures and/or pulmonary vascular resistance in patients with severe functional TR (class IIb) [19].

The lack of evidence on this topic warrants a reasoned approach to drug treatment, informed by pathophysiological considerations. Specific recommendations exist for two possible etiologies of TR, i.e., infective endocarditis and acute pulmonary embolism; the interested reader is reminded to dedicated Guidelines [20, 21].

Medical therapy of TR may be either symptomatic or target the underlying disorder. The following goals must be pursued:

1) treating dysfunctional ventricle(s) through drugs acting on neurohormonal imbalance or inotropes;
2) reducing pulmonary and/or peripheral congestion through diuretics, while avoiding RV underfilling;
3) relieving pulmonary hypertension.

Treating Dysfunctional Ventricle(s)

RV failure can derive from many causes, including pulmonary hypertension, myocardial or pericardial disorders, or RV ischemia. In case of acute RV failure, dysfunction rapidly progresses in geometry alterations and contraction reduction, the RV becomes more spherical and TR develops [22]. In this setting, therapy is based on diuretics and vasopressors and/or on cautious volume expansion through Saline or Ringer lactate (to avoid RV underfilling) [23].

The failing RV undergoes remodeling marked by alterations in expression of a fetal gene program including increased expression of phosphodiesterase-5 (PDE-5), especially in patients with ischemic cardiomyopathy [24]. PDE-5 inhibitors can increase RV inotropy independent of concurrent reduction of RV outflow impedance [25]. However, when TR is complicated by RV failure, the clinical benefit of PDE-5 inhibitors remains to be demonstrated.

The cornerstone of treatment for chronic HF due to LV failure is represented by neurohormonal antagonism with beta-blockers, and mineralocorticoid receptor antagonists (MRA), angiotensin-converting enzyme inhibitors (ACEi), angiotensin-receptor blockers (ARB) or the neprilysin inhibitor -angiotensin receptor blocker sacubitril-valsartan, which improve myocardial function and have a positive impact on the natural history of the disease. Diuretics may be added to relieve congestion. Ivabradine may be added for patients on sinus rhythm and heart rate >70 b.p.m. despite beta-blocker therapy. In the absence of specific evidence, Guideline recommendations for chronic LV failure with reduced ejection fraction apply also to biventricular or isolated RV failure [26, 27].

Reducing Pulmonary and Peripheral Congestion and Avoiding Right Ventricular Underfilling

Furosemide and the other loop diuretics promote diuresis and natriuresis by acting on the renal Na-K-Cl cotransporter. These drugs also inhibit the same cotransporter in the alveoli, likely favoring fluid clearance from the lungs [28], and induce a prostaglandin-dependent venodilation that reduces RV preload [29].

Elevated central venous pressure may cause renal congestion, manifesting as reduced kidney perfusion and glomerular filtration rate [30]. Renal function may be further depressed by sympathetic and renin-angiotensin-aldosterone system (RAAS) activation secondary to HF [31]. Diuretic resistance can derive also from nephron remodeling, with hypertrophy of the distal convolute tubule and increased ion reabsorption [32]. Abnormalities in plasma electrolytes or albumin or therapy with nonsteroidal anti-inflammatory drugs may also promote diuretic resistance. In all these instances, diuretic uptitration may be required [33]. The efficacy of different non-pharmacological therapies for refractory edema (e.g., ultrafiltration) has not been proven in the setting of severe TR.

In patients with TR secondary to LV failure, ACEi/ARB may reduce congestion by improving cardiac output and renal function. Sacubitril-valsartan exerts also an inhibitory effect on neprilysin, thus inhibiting natriuretic peptide degradation; for this reason, sacubitril-valsartan should be even more effective in relieving congestion in this setting, although this point has never been specifically assessed. MRA provide a complementary approach to loop diuretics in patients with refractory congestion [34], as suggested also by ESC HF Guidelines [26].

Morphine, vasodilators (such as nitroglycerin or nitroprusside) and inotropes (dobutamine and also digoxin) have been shown to reduce pulmonary congestion in studies on acute HF with pulmonary edema [29]. These approaches may be considered when TR is associated to these conditions.

As stated above, it is important to remind that an excessive reduction of central venous pressure may worsen RV function because of the Frank-Starling mechanism, resulting in pulmonary hypoperfusion and LV underfilling [35]. Although no specific evidence from published studies is available, maintaining a RV diastolic filling pressure of 8-12 mmHg is then considered a good target. To achieve this goal, moderate sodium restriction (indicatively 2 g/die) and cautious use of diuretics, nitrates, and other medications reducing RV preload is advisable [27, 36].

RELIEVING PULMONARY HYPERTENSION

AHA Guidelines on valve heart diseases recommend to consider lowering elevated pulmonary artery pressures and/or pulmonary vascular resistances in patients with severe functional TR, with a C level of evidence reflecting the lack of evidence from clinical trials [19].

TR can be secondary to pulmonary hypertension (PH) and can benefit from a reduction of high pulmonary artery pressure [2, 3, 21]. According to latest ESC Guidelines, PH is the condition when mean pulmonary arterial pressure (PAPm) measured by right heart catheterization (RHC) is ≥25 mmHg. PH is defined pre-capillary when pulmonary arterial wedge pressure (PAWP) is ≤15 mmHg and post-capillary with PAWP >15 mmHg. Isolated post-capillary PH is the combination of diastolic pressure gradient (DPR diastolic PAP - mean PAWP) <7 mmHg and/or pulmonary vascular resistances (PVR) ≤3 Wood Units (WU). Combined post-capillary and pre-capillary PH is present when DPG is ≥7 mmHg and/or PVR are >3 WU [21]. PH also is also classified according to its etiology into the following groups: 1 (pulmonary arterial hypertension - PAH), 2 (PH due to left heart disease), 3 (PH due to chronic lung disease and/or hypoxemia), 4 (PH due to chronic thromboembolism), 5 (PH due to unclear multifactorial mechanisms). This classification and the identification of the underlying disorder are important to inform therapeutic decision. In the specific case of idiopathic, heritable or drug-induced PAH, RHC allows to perform vasoreactivity testing to identify patients who could benefit from high-dose calcium channel blockers, endothelin receptor antagonists, phosphodiesterase type 5 inhibitors and guanylate cyclase stimulators or prostacyclin analogues. Other supportive pharmacological options in patients with PH include diuretics for patients with HF, and anticoagulants for those with chronic thromboembolic PH. In all these instances, the effect of these therapies on TR severity has not been specifically investigated.

Which Role for Drug Therapy in Tricuspid Regurgitation?

When not caused by acute conditions, TR is generally characterized by long asymptomatic phases during which hemodynamic severity may progress. Severe TR leads to RV pressure and volume overload culminating in RV failure, which is a strong predictor of adverse outcome [37].

First-line treatment of severe TR is valve repair or replacement [17, 19]. Contrary to other valve disorders, no rigorous evidence supports pharmacological therapy for TR, although drug therapies may be appropriate in acute TR, or as a bridge to intervention in decompensated patients. Diuretics are recommended for patients with signs of RV failure, but can limit RV preload and then forward output. The only other therapeutic option recommended is the reduction of elevated pulmonary artery pressures and/or pulmonary vascular resistances. Conceptually, the therapeutic goals of medical treatment for TR are treating dysfunctional ventricle(s), reducing pulmonary and/or peripheral congestion while avoiding RV underfilling, and relieving pulmonary hypertension. Strategies to achieve these goals allow symptom control and patient stabilization rather than being disease-modifying therapies, with the possible exception of neurohormonal antagonists. For this reason, medical treatment should not delay surgery to avoid the development of irreversible RV dysfunction. When patients are not candidates to surgery, percutaneous treatment of TR, if feasible, should be preferred over medical therapy alone.

References

[1] Singh JP, Evans JC, Levy D, Larson MG, Freed LA, Fuller DL, Lehman B, Benjamin EJ (1999) Prevalence and clinical determinants of mitral, tricuspid, and aortic regurgitation (The Framingham Heart Study). *Am J Cardiol* 83:897–902.

[2] Glancy DL, Marcus FI, Cuadra M, Ewy GA, Roberts WC (1969) Isolated organic tricuspid valvular regurgitation. *Am J Med* 46:989–996.

[3] Spinner EM, Lerakis S, Higginson J, Pernetz M, Howell S, Veledar E, Yoganathan AP (2012) Correlates of Tricuspid Regurgitation as Determined by 3D Echocardiography: Pulmonary Arterial Pressure, Ventricle Geometry, Annular Dilatation, and Papillary Muscle Displacement. *Circ Cardiovasc Imaging* 5:43–50.

[4] Park Y-H, Song J-M, Lee E-Y, Kim Y-J, Kang D-H, Song J-K (2008) Geometric and hemodynamic determinants of functional

tricuspid regurgitation: a real-time three-dimensional echocardiography study. *Int J Cardiol* 124:160–165.

[5] Ong K, Yu G, Jue J (2014) Prevalence and spectrum of conditions associated with severe tricuspid regurgitation. *Echocardiography* 31:558–562.

[6] Kim H-K, Kim Y-J, Park J-S, Kim KH, Kim K-B, Ahn H, Sohn D-W, Oh B-H, Park Y-B, Choi Y-S (2006) Determinants of the Severity of Functional Tricuspid Regurgitation. *Am J Cardiol* 98:236–242.

[7] Nemoto N, Lesser JR, Pedersen WR, Sorajja P, Spinner E, Garberich RF, Vock DM, Schwartz RS (2015) Pathogenic structural heart changes in early tricuspid regurgitation. *J Thorac Cardiovasc Surg* 150:323–330.

[8] Chan KMJ (2016) Anatomy of the Tricuspid Valve and Pathophysiology of Functional Tricuspid Regurgitation. In: Funct. *Mitral Tricuspid Regurgitation*. Springer International Publishing, pp 157–162.

[9] Arsalan M, Walther T, Smith RL, Grayburn PA (2017) Tricuspid regurgitation diagnosis and treatment. *Eur Heart J* 38:634–638.

[10] Calafiore AM, Gallina S, Iacò AL, Contini M, Bivona A, Gagliardi M, Bosco P, Di Mauro M (2009) Mitral valve surgery for functional mitral regurgitation: should moderate-or-more tricuspid regurgitation be treated? a propensity score analysis. *Ann Thorac Surg* 87:698–703.

[11] Veire NRV de, Braun J, Delgado V, Versteegh MIM, Dion RA, Klautz RJM, Bax JJ (2011) Tricuspid annuloplasty prevents right ventricular dilatation and progression of tricuspid regurgitation in patients with tricuspid annular dilatation undergoing mitral valve repair. *J Thorac Cardiovasc Surg* 141:1431–1439.

[12] Nath J, Foster E, Heidenreich PA (2004) Impact of tricuspid regurgitation on long-term survival. *J Am Coll Cardiol* 43:405–409.

[13] Topilsky Y, Nkomo VT, Vatury O, et al. (2014) Clinical Outcome of Isolated Tricuspid Regurgitation. *JACC Cardiovasc Imaging* 7:1185–1194.

[14] Lee J-W, Song J-M, Park JP, Lee JW, Kang D-H, Song J-K (2010) Long-Term Prognosis of Isolated Significant Tricuspid Regurgitation. *Circ J* 74:375–380.
[15] Lankeit M, Keller K, Tschöpe C, Pieske B (2017) Medikamentöse Therapie der Trikuspidalklappeninsuffizienz. *Herz* 42:634–643.
[16] Andersen MJ, Nishimura RA, Borlaug BA (2014) The Hemodynamic Basis of Exercise Intolerance in Tricuspid Regurgitation. *Circ Heart Fail* 7:911–917.
[17] Baumgartner H, Falk V, Bax JJ, et al. (2017) 2017 ESC/EACTS guidelines for the management of valvular heart disease. *Eur Heart J* 38:2739–2791.
[18] Beckhoff F, Alushi B, Jung C, Navarese E, Franz M, Kretzschmar D, Wernly B, Lichtenauer M, Lauten A (2018) Tricuspid Regurgitation – Medical Management and Evolving Interventional Concepts. *Front Cardiovasc Med.* doi: 10.3389/fcvm.2018.00049.
[19] Nishimura RA, Otto CM, Bonow RO, et al. (2014) 2014 AHA/ACC Guideline for the Management of Patients With Valvular Heart Disease: Executive Summary. *Circulation* 129:2440–2492.
[20] Habib G, Lancellotti P, Antunes MJ, et al. (2015) 2015 ESC Guidelines for the management of infective endocarditis: The Task Force for the Management of Infective Endocarditis of the European Society of Cardiology (ESC). Endorsed by: European Association for Cardio-Thoracic Surgery (EACTS), the European Association of Nuclear Medicine (EANM). *Eur Heart J* 36:3075–3128.
[21] Galie N, Hoeper MM, Humbert M, et al. (2009) Guidelines for the diagnosis and treatment of pulmonary hypertension: The Task Force for the Diagnosis and Treatment of Pulmonary Hypertension of the European Society of Cardiology (ESC) and the European Respiratory Society (ERS), endorsed by the International Society of Heart and Lung Transplantation (ISHLT). *Eur Heart J* 30:2493–2537.
[22] Harjola V-P, Mebazaa A, Čelutkien\.e J, et al. (2016) Contemporary management of acute right ventricular failure: a statement from the Heart Failure Association and the Working Group on Pulmonary

Circulation and Right Ventricular Function of the European Society of Cardiology. *Eur J Heart Fail* 18:226–241.

[23] Haddad F, Hunt SA, Rosenthal DN, Murphy DJ (2008) Right ventricular function in cardiovascular disease, part I: Anatomy, physiology, aging, and functional assessment of the right ventricle. *Circulation* 117:1436–1448.

[24] Shan X, Quaile MP, Monk JK, French B, Cappola TP, Margulies KB (2012) Differential Expression of PDE5 in Failing and Nonfailing Human Myocardium. *Circ Heart Fail* 5:79–86.

[25] Nagendran J, Archer SL, Soliman D, et al. (2007) Phosphodiesterase type 5 is highly expressed in the hypertrophied human right ventricle, and acute inhibition of phosphodiesterase type 5 improves contractility. *Circulation* 116:238–248.

[26] Ponikowski P, Voors AA, Anker SD, et al. (2016) 2016 ESC Guidelines for the diagnosis and treatment of acute and chronic heart failure: The Task Force for the diagnosis and treatment of acute and chronic heart failure of the European Society of Cardiology (ESC). Developed with the special contribution of the Heart Failure Association (HFA) of the ESC. *Eur J Heart Fail* 18:891–975.

[27] Yancy CW, Jessup M, Bozkurt B, et al. (2013) 2013 ACCF/AHA guideline for the management of heart failure: a report of the American College of Cardiology Foundation/American Heart Association Task Force on practice guidelines. *Circulation* 128:e240-327.

[28] Solymosi EA, Kaestle-Gembardt SM, Vadasz I, et al. (2013) Chloride transport-driven alveolar fluid secretion is a major contributor to cardiogenic lung edema. *Proc Natl Acad Sci* 110:E2308–E2316.

[29] Chioncel O, Collins SP, Ambrosy AP, Gheorghiade M, Filippatos G (2015) Pulmonary Oedema-Therapeutic Targets. *Card Fail Rev* 1:38–45.

[30] Wencker D (2007) Acute cardio-renal syndrome: Progression from congestive heart failure to congestive kidney failure. *Curr Heart Fail Rep* 4:134–138.

[31] Sarraf M, Masoumi A, Schrier RW (2009) Cardiorenal Syndrome in Acute Decompensated Heart Failure. *Clin J Am Soc Nephrol* 4:2013–2026.

[32] Ellison DH, Felker GM (2017) Diuretic Treatment in Heart Failure. *N Engl J Med* 377:1964–1975.

[33] Sonne C (2016) Diagnostik und konservative Therapie der Trikuspidalklappeninsuffizienz [Diagnosis and conservative therapy of tricuspid valve insufficiency]. *CardioVasc* 16:45–51.

[34] Masoumi A, Ortiz F, Radhakrishnan J, Schrier RW, Colombo PC (2014) Mineralocorticoid receptor antagonists as diuretics: Can congestive heart failure learn from liver failure? *Heart Fail Rev* 20:283–290.

[35] Braunwald NS, Ross JR J, Morrow AG (1967) Conservative management of tricuspid regurgitation in patients undergoing mitral valve replacement. *Circulation* 35:I–63.

[36] Heart Failure Society of America, Lindenfeld J, Albert NM, et al. (2010) HFSA 2010 Comprehensive Heart Failure Practice Guideline. *J Card Fail* 16:e1-194.

[37] Borer JS, Sharma A (2015) Drug Therapy for Heart Valve Diseases: Table. *Circulation* 132:1038–1045.

In: The Rediscovered Tricuspid Valve
Editor: Giacomo Bianchi
ISBN: 978-1-53616-098-7

Chapter 11

TRICUSPID VALVE IN THE FAILING HEART: THE ROLE OF TRICUSPID VALVE DURING MECHANICAL CIRCULATORY SUPPORT AND IN HEART TRANSPLANTATION

Ciro Mastroianni[1], MD, PhD, Antonio Nenna[1], MD, Mariafrancesca Fiorentino[2], MD, Sofia Martin-Suarez[2], MD, Massimo Chello[1], MD, and Antonio Loforte[2,*], MD, PhD

[1]Cardiovascular Surgery, Università Campus Bio-Medico, Rome, Italy
[2]Cardiothoracic, Transplantation and Vascular Surgery, S. Orsola Hospital, University of Bologna, Bologna, Italy

ABSTRACT

Tricuspid regurgitation (TR) plays a pivotal role in both short-term and long-term outcomes in patients with advanced heart failure

* Corresponding Author's E-mail: antonioloforte@yahoo.it.

undergoing left ventricular assist device (LVAD) implantation or heart transplantation (HTx). A concomitant tricuspid valve procedure at the time of LVAD implantation might be useful to address moderate-to-severe TR and dilated tricuspid annulus and should be preferably performed with annuloplasty ring. Considering long-term outcomes, tricuspid repair is durable after 1 year and may provide long-term clinical benefits in patients with significant TR. In HTx, TR might be present in donor heart or might develop after procedure. In case of refractory symptoms, surgical treatment should be considered, and the operative approach should be tailored to the underlying mechanisms of TR. In case of anatomic TR (related to endomyocardial biopsies), valve replacement should be preferred, and a biological prosthesis appears reasonable in all patients. In case of functional TR with isolated tricuspid annular dilation, tricuspid valve annuloplasty might be adequate only in selected patients, as pulmonary hypertension and right ventricular failure may result in recurrent TR after repair, and a prosthesis might be the optimal solution. Strategies to reduce the incidence and the clinical impact of TR at time of HTx include the use of bicaval technique and tension-free anastomoses. Concomitant tricuspid valve annuloplasty at the time of HTx might be considered in selected cases. However, there is insufficient information to draw definitive conclusions on the impact of tricuspid valve surgery on postoperative outcomes and further data are needed to choose wisely the best practice for these critically-ill patients.

Keywords: tricuspid valve, tricuspid regurgitation, heart transplantation, left ventricular assist device, right heart failure

INTRODUCTION

Refractory heart failure (HF) unresponsive to medical therapy can be treated with left ventricular assist device or heart transplantation. Tricuspid regurgitation (TR) is common in patients with advanced HF and results from progressive right ventricular (RV) and tricuspid annular dilatation in response to pulmonary venous hypertension from left-sided heart disease. In patients undergoing left ventricular assist device (LVAD), this functional TR has a prevalence of about 50% [1], but whether TR should be surgically managed at the time of LVAD implantation is greatly debated. On the other hand, the number of heart transplantation (HTx) performed annually worldwide has remains static at approximately 4000, and the median survival of 11 years following HTx has remained stable throughout time. Tricuspid valve regurgitation in the donor allograft is the most common valvular complication after HTx, with a reported incidence of up to 84% [2, 3]. The role of tricuspid valve is being increasingly acknowledged as a determinant of perioperative and long-term outcomes, and this chapter will summarize mechanism, prognostic impact and surgical strategies on tricuspid valve in patients undergoing LVAD implantation and HTx.

METHODS

Randomized controlled trials, observational and retrospective studies evaluating LVAD alone versus LVAD plus tricuspid valve surgery (repair or replacement) were considered. On December 2018, SCOPUS, Web of Science, Ovid EMBASE and PubMed/Medline were searched using the following terms and their MeSH analogues: "LVAD" or "ventricular assist device" AND "tricuspid" or "tricusp*." Abstract were identified, and full text articles were reviewed to determine the final studies eligible for inclusion. Our search strategy identified 16 relevant publications [6, 9-11, 13, 15, 17-26] [4–21]. After articles evaluation, references were checked for other potential publications. Summary of the main comparative studies evaluating the effect of TV surgery at the time of LVAD implantation are shown in Table 1.

IMPACT OF TRICUSPID VALVE SURGERY ON LEFT VENTRICULAR ASSIST DEVICE INSERTION

Postoperative RV failure occurs in 40-65% of patients after LVAD implantation [22], requiring prolonged Intensive Care Unit (ICU) stay, implantation of right ventricular assist device (RVAD) or experiencing increased mortality [23]. The presence of preoperative TR is associated with increased postoperative RV failure after LVAD implantation [1].

Occurrence of severe RV failure is one risk factor for peri- and post-operative mortality and morbidity in patients undergoing LVAD implantation, with a reported incidence of 20-40%, and generally requiring device therapy [15].

Among patients undergoing LVAD implantation, 10-15% require implantation of an RVAD [15, 23]. Prediction and treatment of RV failure are important to improve survival after LVAD implantation. Kormos et al. showed that the tricuspid valve (TV) stroke work index and the ratio of central venous pressure and pulmonary capillary wedge pressure are critical predictors of RV failure after LVAD and that RV failure significantly reduced survival after LVAD implantation [23]. Functional TR is common in patients with RV failure and the presence of TR in the setting of RV failure is associated with a poor prognosis [7, 15, 24].

The surgical correction of TR at the time of LVAD implantation might improve RV function and therefore LVAD flow but considering lack of updated and systematically published data this indication remains operator-dependent [1, 6, 9-12, 15, 18, 20, 21, 25]. Some surgeons prefer aggressive approach for tricuspid valve repair (considering a moderate-to-severe TR as a general indication) [21], while other prefer to avoid concomitant tricuspid valve procedure to shorten cardiopulmonary bypass time [20]. TR might not be treated because of concerns that acute increase in TV afterload which occurs when the tricuspid valve is made competent would precipitate worsening or intractable RV failure [6]. Also, after left ventricular (LV) unloading from LVAD, the leftward shift of the interventricular septum results in changes of the geometry of the RV that might cause tricuspid annulus distortion, worsening TR and RV function [17, 26]. Moreover, the regurgitant tricuspid flow might reduce antegrade flow through the pulmonary circulation thus reducing LV preload and LVAD flows [1]. Significant volume-loading and transfusion requirements that are often necessary in the postoperative period may also exacerbate TR when flows are limited by output across the pulmonary vascular bed [17]. Non-regression or progression of TR can have implications in terms of perioperative course, worsening symptoms and functional outcome [4, 6]. Due to prolonged back-pressure changes and congestive hepatomegaly, these patients tend to be more coagulopathic, and therefore relieving afterload on venous return improves hepatic function and thus coagulopathy [6]. This might reduce blood transfusion and its known complications, such as infections, increased pulmonary vascular resistance and allosensitization. Reduced transfusion-related volume requirements may also reduce chances of RV failure due to volume overload in the need for RVAD. In patients receiving LVAD as a destination therapy, persisting TR can implicate persisting symptoms of HF, thus limiting the benefits of device therapy in the long term. It could be possible to argue that, in patients with significant TR undergoing LVAD placement, who are expected to be supported for long periods, restoring annular size and geometry of the tricuspid valve and apparatus should be undertaken as it would improve the symptomatic and prognostic benefits of LVAD placement [6].

Tricuspid Regurgitation at the Time of LVAD Implant and Current Scenario

Data from Interagency Registry for Mechanically Assisted Circulatory Support (INTERMACS) indicate that TR at the time of LVAD implant was extremely common [21]. Among 2527 patients, severe (N=266, 10.5%) and moderate (N=723, 28.6%) TR accounted for more than a third of overall patients undergoing LVAD implantation. Patients with significant TR were not uniformly treated with TV procedure at the time of LVAD implant. Even among patients with severe TR, 35.5% (N=94) underwent TV repair, 3.0% underwent TV replacement (N=8) and 61.7% (N=164) had no procedure. Among patients with moderate TR, 82.0% (N=593) underwent no concomitant valve procedure. Considerable variation in the use of concomitant TV surgery was observed among higher-volume INTERMACS centers, as centers with at least 20 patients with moderate or severe TR at the time of implant were noted to have higher rates of TV surgery [21].

Short Term Outcomes

The single largest published study is a STS database analysis by Robertson et al., who found that performing TV repair failed to reduce early mortality or subsequent RVAD requirement, but significantly increases the risk for postoperative renal failure, greater transfusion requirement, reoperation, prolonged ventilation, prolonged ICU stay and prolonged hospital stay. Their data suggest that additional criteria should be identified to select patients who may benefit from concomitant TV procedures [17].

The only published metanalysis [1] of six observational studies [6, 7, 9, 11, 16, 17] summarized the impact of TV surgery on early postoperative outcomes in 3249 patients. Addition of TV surgery prolonged cardiopulmonary bypass time by an average of 31 minutes (95% CI 20-42 minutes). There was no difference in need for RVAD (hazard ratio 1.42, 95% CI 0.54-3.76), acute renal failure (hazard ratio 1.07, 95% CI 0.55-2.10), or early mortality (hazard ratio 1.28, 95% CI 0.78-2.08). Also, no differences in hospital length of stay was observed. Based on this analysis of the literature, TV surgery prolongs cardiopulmonary bypass times but does not significantly affect other postoperative outcomes. However, this meta-analysis [1] includes also studies with cumulative outcomes of multiple concurrent valve surgery [16] which might negatively influence endpoints. Also, this study does not include more recent papers [10, 12–15, 18, 20, 21] and requires an update to confirm those findings, but taken singularly those study support the aforementioned conclusions. In general, a tendency towards longer operation time, longer duration of ICU stay, longer inotropic support, longer duration of mechanical circulatory support are reported in various studies [9, 18], with no benefit regarding right HF or early mortality [7, 9, 17, 18].

Table 1. Summary of the main comparative studies evaluating the effect of tricuspid valve surgery at time of LVAD implantation

Study	Year	Patients	TVS details	LVAD details	Preoperative differences	Associated procedures	Cardiopulmonary bypass time
Saeed et al. [9]	2011	34 no-TVS 8 TVS	8 repairs (De Vega, ring)	provided	no differences	not reported	CPB time, median TVS: 162 (107-224) min no-TVS: 92 (77-106) min ($P<0.01$)
Piacentino et al. [7]	2011	81 no-TVS 34 TVS	29 repairs (ring) 5 replacements	not provided	TVS: higher central venous pressure / pulmonary capillary wedge pressure ratio	not reported	not reported
Krishan et al. [6]	2012	14 no-TVS 37 TVS	37 repairs (ring)	provided	no differences	TVS: 7 (18.9%) no-TVS: 3 (21.4%) ($P=0.84$)	CPB time, median TVS: 97 min no-TVS: 74 min ($P=0.15$)
Maltais et al. [11]	2012	49 no-TVS 34 TVS	28 repairs (Kay, De Vega, ring) 6 replacements	provided	TVS: more women, more NYHA class IV, more previous sternotomy, more IABP, increased Kormos score, reduced LV systolic diameter, increased RV diastolic and systolic area	not reported	CPB time TVS: 115.8±30.9 min no-TVS: 94.4±33.6 min ($P=0.006$)
Piacentino et al. [8]	2012	28 no-TVS 33 TVS	29 repairs (ring) 4 replacements	provided	no differences	TVS: 18 (54.5%) no-TVS: 19 (67.8%) ($P=0.4$)	CPB time TVS: 179 min no-TVS: 111 ($P<0.001$)
Brewer et al. [14]	2014	87 no-TVS 14 TVS	14 repairs (ring)	provided	TVS: lower body mass index, lower serum glutamic pyruvic transaminase value	not reported	not reported

Table 1. (Continued)

Study	Year	Patients	TVS details	LVAD details	Preoperative differences	Associated procedures	Cardiopulmonary bypass time
Robertson et al. [17]	2014	1608 no-TVS 588 TVS	557 repairs (ring ± reconstruction) 31 replacements	provided	TVS: higher creatinine, lower hypertension, lower dyslipidemia, lower left main disease, lower peripheral vascular disease, lower myocardial infarction, lower moderate-to-severe mitral regurgitation, higher IABP, time-span variations	TVS: 165 (28.1%) no-TVS: 316 (19.7%) (P<0.001)	CPB time TVS: 125.0±42.2 min no-TVS: 88.8±40.2 (P<0.001) AXC time TVS: 59.6±40.6 min no-TVS: 47.8±40.5 (P=0.045)
Oezpeker et al. [18]	2015	26 no-TVS 32 TVS	32 repairs (ring)	not provided	TVS: higher incidence of DCM, lower incidence of ischemic cardiomyopathy, higher dose of epinephrine, lower rate of preop mechanical ventilatory support	TVS: 17 (53.1%) no-TVS: 15 (57.7%) (P=0.728)	CPB time TVS: 136±45 min no-TVS: 104±55 min (P=0.019) AXC time: not provided
Han et al. [20]	2016	252 no-TVS 76 TVS	68 repairs (ring) 8 replacements	provided	TVS: higher central venous pressure, higher total bilirubin., lower hemoglobin	TVS: 35 (46.1%) no-TVS: 114 (45.2%) (P=0.90)	CPB time TVS: 136±52 min no-TVS: 84±39 min (P<0.001) AXC time TVS: 29.0±18.5 min no-TVS: 28.4±11.5 (P=0.86)
Saeed et al. [9]	TVS: 13% no-TVS: 0% (P=0.19)	not reported	TVS: 25% no-TVS: 21% (P=n.s.)	TVS: 3 (38%) no-TVS: 3 (9%) (P=0.07)	not reported	hospital stay, reported as median an interquartile range, in hours TVS: 359 (116-503) no-TVS: 167 (116-252) (P=0.3)	TVS: 1 (13%) no-TVS: 3 (9%) (P=0.6)

Study	Stroke	Dialysis	Reoperation for bleeding	RV failure	Duration of inotropic support	Length of stay	In-hospital mortality	Late outcomes
Saeed et al. [9]	TVS: 13% no-TVS: 0% (P=0.19)	not reported	TVS: 25% no-TVS: 21% (P=n.s.)	TVS: 3 (38%) no-TVS: 3 (9%) (P=0.07)	not reported	hospital stay, reported as median an interquartile range, in hours TVS: 359 (116-503) no-TVS: 167 (116-252) (P=0.3)	TVS: 1 (13%) no-TVS: 3 (9%) (P=0.6)	Saeed et al. [9]
Piacentino et al. [7]	not reported	not reported	not reported	reported as RVAD implantation TVS: 3% no-TVS: 10% (P=0.27)	reported as median an interquartile range, in days TVS: 8 (7-12) no-TVS: 10 (8-17) (P=0.04)	hospital stay, reported as median an interquartile range, in days TVS: 19 (14-25) no-TVS: 26 (16-46) (P=0.02)	not reported	similar survival, not analytically compared
Krishan et al. [6]	not reported	not reported	TVS: 2.7% no-TVS: 7.1% (P=0.44)	not reported	not reported	ICU stay (days, median): TVS 6, no-TVS 5, (P=0.12) Hospital stay (days, median): TVS 18, no-TVS 20, (P=0.42)	TVS: 7 (18.9%) no-TVS: 2 (14.2%) (P=0.70)	not reported
Maltais et al. [11]	TVS: 5 (15%) no-TVS: 4 (8%) (P=0.32)	TVS: 18% no-TVS: 7% (P=0.16)	not reported	TVS: 26% no-TVS: 36% (P=0.51)	TVS: 207±286 hours no-TVS: 191±270 hours (P=0.80)	TVS: 23±16 days no-TVS: 20±12 days (P=0.46)	TVS: 17.6% no-TVS: 4.1% (P=0.07)	similar survival (maximum follow up 2.5 years, no mode details provided) (P=0.26)

Table 1. (Continued)

Study	Stroke	Dialysis	Reoperation for bleeding	RV failure	Duration of inotropic support	Length of stay	In-hospital mortality	Late outcomes
Piacentino et al. [8]	not reported	not reported	not reported	TVS: 6 (18.2%) no-TVS: 13 (46.4%) (P<0.05)	TVS: 9.7 days no-TVS: 12.1 days (P=0.16)	reported as patients requiring more than 30 days of hospitalization TVS: 6/33 (18.2%) no-TVS: 12/28 (42.9%) (P<0.05) reported as median and interquartile range TVS: 19 (13-27) days no-TVS: 20 (15-37) days (P=0.21)	TVS: 1 (3.1%) no-TVS: 1 (3.5%) (P=1.0)	1-year survival TVS: 21/24 (87.5%) no-TVS: 17/22 (77.3%) (P=0.45)
Brewer et al. [14]	not reported	not reported	TVS: 2 (14.3%) no-TVS: 17 (19.5%) (P=n.s.)	TVS: 4 (28.6%) no-TVS: 12 (13.8%) (P=0.43)	not reported	not reported	TVS: 1 (7.1%) no-TVS: 11 (12.6%) (P=n.s.)	not reported
Robertson et al. [17]	events: 67/2153 (3.1%) risk ratio for TVS (after PS-IPW): 0.65 (95% CI 0.32-1.33, P=0.24)	events: 155/2088 (7.4%) risk ratio for TVS (after PS-IPW): 1.49 (95% CI 1.03-2.15, P=0.034)	events: 345/2154 (16.0%) risk ratio for TVS (after PS-IPW): 1.16 (95% CI 0.89-1.51, P=0.26)	reported as RVAD implantation events: 98/2161 (4.5%) risk ratio for TVS (after PS-IPW): 0.81 (95% CI 0.49-1.36, P=0.43)	not reported	after PS-IPW ICU stay (hours): TVS 303.2, no-TVS 294.5, mean difference 8.6 (P=0.62) Hospital stay (days): TVS 29.4, no-TVS 25.8, mean difference 3.6 (P=0.083)	events: 221/2161 (10.2%) risk ratio for TVS (after PS-IPW): 0.95 (95% CI 0.68-1.33, P=0.766)	not reported

Study	Stroke	Dialysis	Reoperation for bleeding	RV failure	Duration of inotropic support	Length of stay	In-hospital mortality	Late outcomes
Oezpeker et al. [18]	not reported	TVS: 12 (37.5%) no-TVS: 7 (26.9%) (P=0.761)	TVS: 11 (34.4%) no-TVS: 9 (34.6%) (P=0.727)	TVS: 23 (71.9%) no-TVS: 16 (61.5%) (P=0.29)	TVS: 34.8±35.9 days no-TVS: 19.0±14.3 days (P=0.040)	ICU stay (days): TVS 46.4±50.7, no-TVS 24.5±22.1, (P=0.045) Hospital stay (days): TVS 63.1±54.9, no-TVS 51.6±28.0, (P=0.337)	TVS: 2 (6.3%) no-TVS: 1 (3.9%) (P=0.530)	1-year survival: TVS 53.1%, no-TVS 73.1% (P=0.176). Propensity-score adjusted mortality risk for TVS: 3.05 (95% CI 0.8-11.1, P=0.091).
Han et al. [20]	TVS: 5 (6.6%) no-TVS: 18 (7.2%) (P=0.85)	TVS: 14 (18.9%) no-TVS: 37 (15.1%) (P=0.43)	TVS: 19 (27.5%) no-TVS: 38 (16.7%) (P=0.046)	TVS: 16 (21%) no-TVS: 68 (27%) (P=0.95)	not reported	ICU stay (days): TVS 11.0±10.2, no-TVS 10.0±10.6, (P=0.44) Hospital stay (days): TVS 40.6±50.2, no-TVS 35.0±31.1, (P=0.25)	TVS: 8 (10.5%) no-TVS: 16 (6.4%) (P=0.22)	2-year survival: TVS 73.9%, no-TVS 74.2% (P=0.24) readmission (average cumulative events at 2 years): TVS 2.16, no-TVS 1.60 (P=0.091)

Echocardiography results show the immediate and continuous benefit of TV procedure on reducing TR. Han et al. evaluated 252 patients undergoing LVAD implantation alone and 76 patients receiving also TV surgery, and in the TV repair group 90% of patients had none-to-mild TR within 1 month after initial discharge [20]. Piacentino et al. showed improvement in TR in patients who underwent LVAD alone and in those with associated TV procedure, but the improvement is more immediate and greater in magnitude for the group that was treated with the concomitant tricuspid procedures; 94% of patients treated with a concomitant procedure had none to mild TR immediately after the procedure; in contrast, 75% of patients treated with LVAD alone remained with moderate or severe TR on the echocardiograms immediately after the procedure [8].

The most probable cause for increased major morbidities is underlying preoperative progressive right HF in patients with significant preoperative TR. Underlying right HF can lead to congestive hepatopathy and impair the synthesis of clotting factors, thus increasing the risk of bleeding and therefore reoperation [5, 20]. Another contributing factor would be risk of bleeding from additional right atriotomy and prolonged cardiopulmonary bypass time [20]. However, TV repair does not take more than 15-20 minutes in experienced hands and could be performed on a beating heart. Therefore, although the duration of CPB is increased in a statistically significant way, this is not likely to be translated in a clinically significant alteration.

TV surgery is also reported to require additional transfusion requirement and increased risk of renal failure [9, 17], but those differences could reflect the effects of the right heart on end-organ function. Also, those complications might be consequences of prolonged cardiopulmonary or cross-clamp time.

With regards to short-term outcomes, the current literature does not report a significant benefit for TV surgery at time of LVAD implantation. However, this could possibly reflect the effectiveness of medial therapy of RV failure with pulmonary vasodilators and inotropic agents. Also, patient selection for concomitant TV surgery failed to identify patients who would benefit from TV repair or replacement due to postoperative exacerbations of RV failure.

Long-Term Outcomes

Considering long-term echocardiographic durability of TV procedures, Han et al. concluded that TV surgery was protective for developing future significant tricuspid regurgitation (odds ratio 0.38, 95% confidence interval 0.19-0.76, p = 0.006), and TV repair has good long-term durability [20]. Another study showed that TR grade was significantly decreased from 2.6 to 1.0 after TV repair, and this decrease was maintained for 2 years [15]. Therefore, concomitant TV repair appears to be a durable procedure for restoring deteriorated RV function.

Significant TR at the time of LVAD implantation was associated with worsened survival at follow up: patients with moderate-to-severe TR had a significantly poorer survival (p=0.009), which was apparent during the entire period of follow up (46 months). Each level of increase in TR (from mild to moderate to severe) has a hazard ratio of 1.35 (p=0.009) for death after LVAD implantation [21].

There have not been enough studies evaluating long-term (> 1 year) effects of TV surgery, and results are conflicting. One report from the HeartMate II trial from the STS database showed 1- and 2-year survivals of 77% and 63%, respectively [17]. Those results are similar to Han et al., with similar long-term outcomes, with 75.2%and 63.7% survivals at 1 and 2 years, respectively; the same author found that, after 2 years of device support, long-term incidences of right HR readmission in patients with TV procedures are not different from LVAD only patients. Patients with moderate TR left untreated had worse on-device survival (76.0%), whereas moderate TR treated with TV procedures showed comparable survival to nonsignificant TR (93.3% vs 92.5%). At the same time, patients with at least moderate-to-severe TR and treated with TV procedure had worse on-device survival compared with the nonsignificant TR group (82.1% vs 92.5%) [20]. In the STS analysis, however, TV repair did not appear to confer a survival benefit among patients with moderate or severe TR at the time of LVAD implant, and the Kaplan-Meier survival curve of patients with moderate or severe TR who underwent TV repair was not superior to that of patients with moderate or severe TR who underwent no TV procedures. The higher frequency of coronary artery disease in the "no TV procedure group" was the only characteristic with a statistically significant difference between the two groups, despite a similar INTERMACS level profile [21]. Another study from Oezpeker et al. evaluated a small cohort of 58 patients with severe TR and concluded that concomitant TV repair tends to increase 1-year mortality; TV surgery has no effect on other endpoints such as recurrent TR grade > 2, right HF, postoperative kidney failure, but was associated with longer operation time and duration of ICU stay and inotropic support. Hemodynamic parameters were superior compared to other studies, thus indicating that only severely ill patients might benefit from TV repair [18].

Although repair is necessary for moderate or greater TR, earlier intervention before TR progresses to severe is needed to improve overall survival. Further studies are needed to better evaluate and understand the long-term implications of performing TV surgery at the time of LVAD implantation. However, TV repair appears reasonable and should be considered especially in patients in whom LVAD is used as a destination therapy or a long period on device therapy is estimated. The increasing use of LVAD as a destination therapy underlines the importance of evaluating this issue, as the LVAD remains in situ for the rest of patient's life and the impact of TR might have a profound significance for medical therapy, symptoms and quality of life.

Alternative Echocardiographic Measures

The severity of functional TR can be highly variable thus complicating its diagnosis and the relative treatment. The TR grade depends on volume status and hemodynamics [19, 25]. In patients with volume overload, significant TR might be observed even in the absence of annular dilation, which complicates the assessment of underlying RV function [25]. Tricuspid annular dilation has been suggested as a more reliable marker of concomitant advanced RV failure than severity of TR, and tricuspid annular dilation may represent an initial phase of RV compromise in which TR may or may not be present [27, 28]. Therefore, tricuspid annular dilation might more reliably predict RV failure following LVAD implant [19], and affects long-term survival after LVAD in the absence of TR [29].

Recently, Goldraich et al. found that tricuspid annular dilation (indexed tricuspid annular diameter ≥ 23 mm/m2) was a predictor of postoperative RV failure; greater indexed tricuspid annular dimension was associated with increased duration of inotropic support, suggesting a progressively higher risk of postoperative RV impairment with increasing tricuspid annular diameter [19]. Kukucka et al. identified that a tricuspid annular diameter > 43 mm predicted 3-year mortality after LVAD among a cohort of 122 patients without severe TR [29]. Significant TR that remains or worsens after LVAD implantation might be related to the development of late onset RV failure; in this sense, tricuspid annular dimension might improve risk stratification for RV failure in both early and late postoperative periods, warranting more aggressive use of RIVAD or more appropriate use of surgical techniques to preserve RV function [19]. Tricuspid annular dilation might play a role in the outcome of patients undergoing LVAD implantation regardless the severity of TR [17], and tailored studies are warranted to elucidate this mechanism.

Surgical Approaches

The use of LVAD systems is a life-saving treatment which also provides long-term survival with good quality of life for patients with refractory heart failure. In this setting, right heart function becomes the key to patient's survival, and RV failure remains a significant postoperative complication of LVAD that affects mortality. RV failure is known to reduce 1-year survival rate from 91% to 65%, 2-year survival rate from 83% to 43% and was shown to be an independent risk factor for long-term survival [15]. Previously, the mechanisms of postoperative RV failure were explained by acute unloading of the LV which leads to a septal shift that alters RV shape and function, thereby affecting contractility; underlying RV impairment has also been reported to be unmasked with increased RV preload [15, 30, 31]. TR is common in patients with advanced heart failure, occurring as a result of progressive tricuspid annular enlargement and TV leaflet tethering related to progressive RV enlargement that result from RV pressure or volume overload [15]. The development of TR leads to a vicious cycle of progressive RV enlargement and worsening regurgitation. The prevalence of moderate-to-severe TR has been estimated to be nearly 50% among patients undergoing LVAD implantation [8, 11]. Whether TR is treated with tricuspid valve repair or replacement at the time of LVAD implantation depends on the preference of the individual surgeon rather than objective guidelines due to lacks in literature evidences. On one hand, there is concern that fixing the TV may result in progressive RV dysfunction and failure in the early postoperative period. In this context, tricuspid valve function depends on left ventricular function and effective unloading of the LV with an LVAD can determine an improvement in TV function, with a reduced degree of TR [12, 32, 33]. On the other hand, TR has been identified as a predictor of adverse postoperative outcomes [34] and some surgeons repair the TV at the time of LVAD implantation in the hope of improving postoperative outcomes and potentially eliminating the need for future tricuspid procedures. Factors that may contribute to resolution of TR in these patients include etiology of heart failure, the degree of LV unloading by the LVAD, pulmonary vascular resistance, RV size and function, and renal function [21], and how these factors interact to cause progressive TV failure and TR is critical to being able to model or predict which subgroups of patients may benefit from a TV procedure.

In the vast majority of the published literature [25], TV surgery is performed for moderate-to-severe TR, with ring annuloplasty being the procedure of choice; in case of severe leaflet tethering or destruction, TV replacement can be performed with a bioprosthetic valve. Deo et al. reported that the choice to repair or replace does not affect the clinical outcomes despite CPB time was longer for patients undergoing TV replacement [10]. However, Jang et al. stated that, compared with TV repair, replacement was associated with higher operative mortality and worse long-term clinical outcomes in patients with very severe functional TR, and authors concluded that TV repair should be the preferred surgical option even for severe TR associated with more advanced tethering and right ventricular dilatation [35]. Therefore, TV repair remains the preferable option when anatomically feasible considering the beneficial effects in RV dynamics. Other centers report the feasibility of De Vega annuloplasty, showing optimal short term and long term results: at 1-year follow up, 90.6% of patients had mild TR, and TV repair failure (recurrent moderate-to-severe TR) was observed in 9.4% of patients [13]. De Vega annuloplasty might potentially reduce cardiopulmonary bypass time and shorter operative time compared to other ring annuloplasty technique and provide satisfactory results. However, in conventional cardiac operations, De Vega TV repair had significantly inferior durability compared to ring annuloplasty [36, 37], but the peculiar hemodynamic changes related to LVAD implantation might improve long-term outcomes, although other studies reported that De Vega technique remains a less effective repair strategy also in LVAD setting [7, 9]. Future studies are warranted to compare those techniques and provide comparable results and definitive indications [25].

Recently, transcatheter tricuspid valve intervention (TTVI) for native tricuspid valve dysfunction has been emerging during the last few years as an alternative therapeutic option to serve a large high-risk population of patients with severe symptomatic tricuspid regurgitation [38, 39]. Results from the TriValve registry indicate that TTVI is feasible with different technologies, has a reasonable overall procedural success rate, and is associated with low mortality and significant clinical improvement, with favorable mid-term survival in high-risk population [40]. Greater coaptation depth is associated with reduced procedural success, which is an independent predictor of mortality [40, 41]. Further studies will evaluate this promising technique in the setting of TR after LVAD implantation [42].

Impact of Tricuspid Valve Surgery on Heart Transplantation

Orthotopic heart transplantation (HTx) remains the gold standard therapy for advanced HF refractory to medical and device management. Tricuspid valve regurgitation in the donor allograft is the most common valvular complication after HTx, with a reported incidence of up to 84% [2, 3], although the high diagnostic rate might reflect a liberal application of the diagnostic criteria towards a dynamic process. While most of TR after HTx is mild and clinically insignificant, approximately one third of patients have moderate-to-severe TR resulting in symptoms such as peripheral edema and dyspnea, resulting in reduced quality of life [3, 43]. A small percentage (about 5%) of patients, however, develop refractory symptoms and surgical correction is warranted with a subsequent procedure [44], and this redo procedure carries an extremely high mortality rate which might be greater than 60% [45]. Increased episodes of acute rejection were correlated to increased TR due to mechanisms of papillary muscle edema and asymmetric contractility of the RV [3, 46]. Despite the resolution of rejection episodes, significant TR increased over time with an incidence of 38% at 1 year and of 62% at 2 years. Over time, the pressure or volume overload can lead to worsening RV function with a reduced cardiac output that can be difficult to distinguish from acute rejection. A recent study confirmed that moderate-to-severe is associated with an increased risk of death, transplant or reoperation [47]. TR might be a coexisting pathology in the donor heart or can develop after HTx, and there are various mechanisms which lead to TR which should be adequately diagnosed and managed to optimize survival.

TR in the Donor Heart and Its Concomitant Treatment

The presence of intraoperative moderate-to-severe negatively impacts long term survival, and a retrospective analysis demonstrated significantly decreased survival for patients with mild or greater (2+ to 4+) TR detected by transesophageal echocardiography at the time of transplantation and RV dysfunction; concomitant TV surgery with annuloplasty has been advocated at time of HTx to improve outcomes in those patients [48].

Brown et al. pioneered that prophylactic TV annuloplasty with either a De Vega or ring technique reduced the incidence of moderate-to-severe early TR [49].

Subsequently, Jeevanandam et al. compared outcomes of patients receiving bicaval HTx with or without concomitant TV repair with De Vega technique in 60 randomized patients [50]. TV annuloplasty was performed on the donor heart before implantation using pledgeted 2-0 polypropylene and sized to an annulus of 29 mm. Patients receiving HTx with concomitant TV repair had improved early survival and better late outcomes, such as cardiac mortality (23% versus 10%), average amount of TR (1.5±1.3 versus 0.5±0.4), patients with 2+ or greater TR (34% versus 0%), serum creatinine (2.9±2.0 versus 1.8±0.7), and difference in serum creatinine over baseline (2.0±2.1 versus 0.7±0.8); the authors concluded that the presence of moderate-to-severe TR requires concomitant treatment at time of HTx to improve short term and long term outcomes and should be considered as a routine procedure [50].

Although De Vega annuloplasty requires on average 7-8 minutes to be performed, its durability has been questioned and annuloplasty ring should be preferred [51]. However, the natural history of TR after HTx remains to be elucidated and recent evidences are pointing out that TR might resolve over time.

A recent study [52] confirmed that significant TR has in incidence of 21% after weaning from CPB with no significant difference in preoperative recipient pulmonary vascular resistance. Significant TR was associated with increased peak postoperative plasma creatinine ($P=0.008$), prolonged postoperative stay (median 12 (9-21) days versus 10 (8-14) days, $P<0.001$), and decreased adjusted survival. Significant TR regressed to insignificant in 91% of recipients by 1-years after HTx, and only 1% of recipients who had significant TR after CPB underwent delayed TV repair for significant TR at follow up. The authors concluded that significant TR is associated with early mortality but the majority of TR resolves by 1 year post-transplant, and optimal algorithms for follow up and treatment of significant TR after HTx need to be clarified.

However, another recent study questioned the efficacy of donor TV repair with an analysis of 330 patients [53], with a De Vega annuloplasty technique over a 26-mm Hegar dilator. Although fewer composite outcomes occurred in the TV repair group (22.5% vs 36.4% in the non-TV repair group, p=0.006), TV repair was not significantly associated with the outcome in multivariable analysis. Lower risk for adverse outcome was associated with greater number of biopsies after 1 year, while higher risk was associated with more high-grade biopsy specimens. In conclusion, there was no significant benefit or harm with regards to the composite of death, post-HTx TR or dialysis.

While TV annuloplasty on the ex vivo heart is relatively a simple procedure with optimal surgical field, is it not universally accepted as standard of care due to lack of consensus regarding definitive benefits outside single center experiences [47, 54, 55] and evidence from recent studies questioning its importance [53, 56].

Etiology of TR after HTx

The prevalence of TR after HTx ranges from 20% to 50-80% [45, 50, 57], depending on the definition of TR and when the diagnosis was made. Mild and moderate tricuspid regurgitation are seen in most the patients, who were responsive to medical therapy and remained clinically stable in NYHA class I-II. Severe tricuspid regurgitation was seen in 10-20% of patients, presenting with signs of an acute right heart dysfunction [54, 57]. Overall, prevalence of moderate-to-severe TR may be as high as 35-40% [43, 54]. TR in the cardiac allograft can have anatomic, functional or infective etiologies.

As far as functional mechanism is concerned, the geometric distortion of the tricuspid annulus and the progressive annular dilation play a pivotal role. In functional TR, the regurgitant jet is typically central and caused by the geometric distortion of the atrioventricular annular ring and dilation, and malcoaptation of the valve leaflets. RV failure can result from high pulmonary vascular resistance, and the RV dilates and increases in length along the superior-inferior axis leading to elliptical/spherical deformation, valvular tethering and coaptation deficit [58]. TV repair or replacement, in this context, alleviate regurgitation but have a small influence on overall RV function. Re-transplantation can hardly be considered an option, as the second heart will behave similarly when faced with elevated pulmonary vascular resistance.

As far as anatomic mechanism is concerned, many studies showed a causal link between the number of endomyocardial biopsies (EMB) and the development of TR, thus introducing the concept of "biopsy-related TR." Chordal damage resulting in leaflet flail has been correlated to the number of procedures [3], and in patients with more than 30 procedures the incidence of severe TR reached 60% [59]. The presence of chordal tissue in myocardial specimens has been found in almost half patients with recently diagnosed TR [60].

Also, a very small percentage of patients might experience endocarditis, which is mainly related to EMB as it increases susceptibility of the damaged valve to bacterial seeding [3]. Other interplaying factors though to influence the occurrence and severity of TR include the technique of allograft implantation [61], frequency of endomyocardial biopsies [60], length of biopsy bioptome sheath [44, 62], ischemic injury to the RV, and size mismatch between the donor heart and pericardial cavity [2, 54].

Impact of Bicaval versus Biatrial Technique at Time of HTx

Shortly after the introduction of bicaval anastomosis technique, there were various single center reports of improved TR over time when compared to standard biatrial technique.

In Laske et al., TR during the first 2 weeks (in 31% of recipients with bicaval and in 70% with atrial anastomoses) improved in all recipients with bicaval anastomoses and in 14% of the recipients with atrial anastomosis, with no differences in CPB time and ischemia time. The authors suggested that the atrioventricular valve function and the postoperative rhythm after orthotopic HTx can be improved by implanting the heart with bicaval anastomoses [63].

In Aziz et al., right atrial pressure and mean pulmonary artery pressure were lower for the bicaval recipients up to 12 months after the operation, while LV ejection fraction was higher for the recipients of the bicaval technique. The prevalence of moderate-to-severe TR was higher in the recipients of the biatrial technique compared to bicaval (28% vs 7%; P =0.02). The actuarial survival at 1, 3, and 5 years was 74%, 70%, and 62% for the recipients of the biatrial technique versus 87%, 82%, and 81% for the recipients of the bicaval technique, which also showed improved survival [64].

Those results were also confirmed by Berger et al. who found that at the end of the follow up (average 8.2 years) significant TR was evident in 14.1% of the patients and the development of late TR was found to be significantly correlated with the biatrial surgical technique ($p < 0.01$) and the presence of graft vasculopathy ($p < 0.001$) [45].

Subsequently, many papers have documented the superiority of the bicaval technique over the biatrial technique for short-term outcomes.

A meta-analysis of 41 papers found significant benefits for early atrial pressure, TR, return to sinus rhythm and even perioperative mortality, despite being technically more demanding and requiring a slightly longer bypass and ischemic time [65]. The enlarged right atrial size of the combined atria in the biatrial technique might exacerbate TR by increasing wall tension and tricuspid annular size during systole [61]. Apart from this anatomic distortion, the biatrial anastomosis might lead to asynchronous atrial contractions with further dilation of the right atrium over time [3].

However, the sole application of bicaval anastomosis is not sufficient to prevent the development and progression of TR, as the generated tension of the bicaval anastomosis might be a risk factor: the stretching of the right atrium might result in tricuspid annulus distortion.

In a small study, augmentation of the inferior vena caval anastomosis with a flap of recipient's atrium leads to a reduction in TR to mild in all patients, but these results were not replicated in larger cohorts [66].

The problem in the current literature remains the study power and sample size, as most studies are underpowered and failed to show durable protection from TR [3].

However, a comprehensive review of the United Network for Organ Sharing failed to show differences in TR outcomes depending on the surgical approach [67]. HTx performed with bicaval anastomoses require postoperative permanent pacemaker implantation at lower frequency (odds ratio for biatrial technique 2.6; 95% confidence interval 2.2-3.1) and have a small but significant survival advantage compared with biatrial anastomoses in both short-term (OR for bicaval technique 0.83; 95% confidence interval 0.75-0.93) and long-term outcomes (HR for biatrial technique 1.11; 95% CI 1.04-1.19), recommending that bicaval anastomoses should be preferred for HTx when technically feasible.

Biopsy Related TR

EMB remains the gold standard of diagnosis and monitoring of acute rejection after HTx, which accounts for approximately 10% of deaths in the first year [68–70].

This procedure has rare but potentially life-threatening complications such as cardiac tamponade or traumatic (anatomic) TR, which occurs in 1% to 4% of patients [71, 72].

Mielniczuk et al. found that histologic evidence of chordal tissue in EMB specimens was present in almost half of patients with significant TR and did not relate to the number of biopsy performed or the frequency of rejection episodes [60].

Williams et al. found that both the prevalence of flail tricuspid leaflet (41% to 6%, $P < 0.0001$) and mean grade of TR (2 to 1, $P < 0.0001$) were reduced after the use of a 45 cm sheath. The authors concluded that TR secondary to biopsy-induced damage to the valve apparatus occurs in cardiac transplant recipients and is associated with signs of early right-sided heart failure, and the use of a 45 cm sheath during EMB reduces the prevalence of flail tricuspid leaflet and the severity of TR [62].

Based on the data of Nguyen et al., despite the lack of current guidelines and the paucity of large registry studies, biopsies should be scheduled and protocolled to a regimen of less than 31 procedures over the lifetime of the allograft to reduce the risk of severe iatrogenic TR [59].

The optimal surgical management of EMB-induced TR is controversial and recent literature seem to point out the beneficial long-term effects of TV replacement over repair. However, recent reports underline the feasibility of repair procedures such as the clover technique [73–75], stitching together with a 5-0 polypropylene suture the middle point of the free edges of the tricuspid leaflets producing a clover-shaped valve, completed with a ring annuloplasty. Midterm clinical and echocardiographic results confirm the role of the 'clover technique' in the surgical treatment of TR due to lesions, which are unlikely to be effectively treatable by annuloplasty alone [76]. The clover technique seems a useful and effective solution in the specific and rare condition of EMB-induced TR as it leads to satisfactory short-term clinical and echocardiographic results. However, further studies are warranted to confirm those findings and compare this approach with TV replacement.

Surgical Approaches

Most patients with TR after HTx do not have enough symptoms to require a surgical procedure and can be treated with diuretics only. However, TR may lead to refractory symptoms and should be treated. Progressive RV enlargement, with disproportionate elongation of the mid-minor axis, elevated right-side pressures and more advanced functional class is a general consequence of moderate-to-severe, hemodynamically significant TR. Up to 75% of patients with TR has overt RV failure in the immediate postoperative period, and this correlated with post-HTx pulmonary hypertension [2]. With longer follow up duration, the severity and clinical impact of TR worsens. TR progression was correlated with changes in RV diastolic area and tricuspid anulus, and intraoperative TR severity is strongly correlated with RV dysfunction, perioperative mortality and late survival [48, 62, 64].

Functional TR, due to tethering mechanisms, might be effectively treated with ring annuloplasty. On the other hand, anatomic TR resulting from chordal or leaflet damage might require valve replacement to avoid suboptimal results after repair. However, about 50% of patients after TV repair might require additional procedures due to recurrent severe TR during follow up.

Alharethi et al.found that TV repair resulted in decreased central venous pressure (mean, from 17.8 mmHg to 11.0 mmHg, p=0.013) and furosemide dose (mean, from 47.7 mg/day to 26.5 mg/day, p=0.009), with no significant change in cardiac output or renal function. Flail leaflets were the most common operative finding, suggesting that biopsy-induced trauma is the likely cause of severe TR in these patients [77].

As size mismatch and operative factors might result in misalignment between right atrium, TV and RV and might determine TR [54], surgical features that might prevent significant TR include matching donor heart size to pericardial cavity size with a reductive pericardial closure, tensionless anastomosis and bicaval technique to maintain native right atrial and RV geometry.

Like native valve disease, indication for surgery should be more imperative in case of an anatomic valvular disease [25]. For functional TR, patients should be carefully selected as pulmonary hypertension, RV failure and TR have a delicate interplay. For instance, patients with a severe RV failure due to fixed pulmonary hypertension are unlikely to have a long-term benefit from TV surgery despite a high perioperative mortality risk. Also, replacement might be favored over repair in case of anatomic disease, e.g., after EMB injury, as replacement is associated with more durable outcomes and improved symptoms [3, 78]. Retrospective studies showed that TV replacement may offer better durability and symptomatic relief for TR after HTx [46, 56, 59, 80] [44, 54, 57, 77]. Surgery to correct severe TR should consider the underlying mechanism.

As EMB remains the gold standard in acute rejection surveillance, tricuspid repair with a downsizing annuloplasty ring may increase the chance of damage to the chordal structures by the bioptome. Therefore, TV repair (with annuloplasty or other procedures) may be more suitable in functional TR where the annulus is dilated initially and where downsizing might restore the normal valve size.

The study from Filsoufi et al. raised concerns about the long-term durability of TV repair, as half procedures failed and required subsequent replacement. If a repair approach is pursued, no more than trivial TR should be intraoperatively accepted as operative goal, and higher grades of TR appear to be at risk of recurrent TR and clinical events [44, 48]. As usual, TV replacement should be performed immediately in case of suboptimal TV repair.

Mechanical valves would not be the wiser choice due to the inability to subsequently perform EMB and the need of anticoagulation [54], while biological valves have excellent long-term durability, do not require anticoagulation and do not pose a contraindication to EMB. Also, a potential subsequent chordal damage during EMB would have no clinical impact, and prosthetic valve leaflet injury is not reported. Some authors suggested that mechanical valves should be considered in patients with chronic renal failure [57], as this would lead to premature calcification and failure of bioprosthesis, and this appears the only possible indication to mechanical TV replacement [25].

Again, transcatheter tricuspid valve intervention (TTVI) could be an interesting operative approach to treat TR in HTx recipients [39, 40, 79]. TTVI in patients with HTx can be a valuable approach to prevent further open-heart surgeries, which carry added morbidity and mortality. Further studies will evaluate this promising technique in the setting of TR after HTx.

Gaps in Evidence

The results of the prophylactic TV repair during HTx suggests that annuloplasty might provide a long-term benefit to HTx recipients by reducing the incidence of TR. However, larger prospective randomized controlled trials are warranted to confirm this strategy. At present, it is not possible to reliably predict which patients with clinically significant TR will improve without the need for surgical intervention, and in which patient the TR will become clinically significant leading to worse outcomesAlso, early postoperative TR might be a marker of graft dysfunction and not necessarily an isolated finding. Alternatives to EMB have been tested, such as AlloMap scores, daily intramyocardial electrocardiography or echocardiographic repeated measures, but EMB remains the gold standard until newer evidences gain enough quality and reach high clinical impact. The results of TV repair in this setting are satisfying in selected cases only (functional TR due to annular dilation), and further studies are required to delineate this potential indication. TV replacement with a bioprosthetic valve seems the most effective treatment to relieve symptoms while facilitating biopsies and allowing further percutaneous valve-in-valve procedures, but larger studies are necessary to provide conclusive evidences.

CONCLUSION

A concomitant TV procedure at the time of LVAD implantation might be useful to address moderate-to-severe TR and dilated tricuspid annulus. TV repair, generally performed using an annuloplasty ring, is the procedure of choice and might reduce TR and positively alter RV geometry, at the cost of a slightly increased cardiopulmonary bypass time. Despite lack of substantial differences in short-term outcomes, at long-term follow up TV repair is durable after 1 year and may provide long-term clinical benefits in patients with significant TR. Therefore, all patients receiving LVAD with significant (moderate-to-severe) TR should be considered for concomitant TV surgery. TV replacement should be considered in the minority of patients, in whom TV apparatus has been damaged and cannot be repaired effectively (e.g., for endocarditic processes). However, there is insufficient information to draw definitive conclusions on the impact of TV surgery on postoperative outcomes and further data are needed to choose wisely the best practice for these critically-ill patients.

TR is a common valvular disease in patients undergoing HTx, and it might be already present in the donor heart or might develop after HTx due to the recipient's pulmonary hemodynamic. In most cases, TR is mild to moderate and could be treated with medical therapy alone to alleviate edema, dyspnea, hepatorenal syndrome and ascites. In case of refractory symptoms, surgical treatment should be considered, and the operative approach should be tailored to the underlying mechanisms of TR and to the specific patient's situation [3]. In case of anatomic TR, valve replacement should be preferred, and a biological prosthesis appears reasonable in all patients. In case of functional TR with isolated tricuspid annular dilation, TV annuloplasty might be adequate only in selected patients, as pulmonary hypertension and RV failure may result in recurrent TR after repair and thus symptoms; most patients can be treated effectively with TV replacement. Strategies to reduce the incidence and the clinical impact of TR at time of HTx include the use of bicaval technique and tension-free anastomoses. Concomitant TV annuloplasty at the time of HTx might be considered in selected cases, and non-invasive surveillance methods are emerging as attractive alternatives to EMB, but further studies are warranted to confirm their clinical effectiveness in clinical practice.

REFERENCES

[1] Dunlay SM, Deo SV, Park SJ (2015) Impact of Tricuspid Valve Surgery at the Time of Left Ventricular Assist Device Insertion on Postoperative Outcomes. *ASAIO J* 61:15–20.

[2] Wong RC-C, Abrahams Z, Hanna M, Pangrace J, Gonzalez-Stawinski G, Starling R, Taylor D (2008) Tricuspid Regurgitation After Cardiac Transplantation: An Old Problem Revisited. *J Heart Lung Transplant* 27:247–252.

[3] Kwon MH, Shemin RJ (2017) Tricuspid valve regurgitation after heart transplantation. *Ann Cardiothorac Surg* 6:270–274.

[4] Anyanwu AC, Chikwe J, Adams DH (2008) Tricuspid valve repair for treatment and prevention of secondary tricuspid regurgitation in patients undergoing mitral valve surgery. *Curr Cardiol Rep* 10:110–117.

[5] Matthews JC, Pagani FD, Haft JW, Koelling TM, Naftel DC, Aaronson KD (2010) Model for End-Stage Liver Disease Score Predicts Left Ventricular Assist Device Operative Transfusion Requirements, Morbidity, and Mortality. *Circulation* 121:214–220.

[6] Krishan K, Nair A, Pinney S, Adams DH, Anyanwu AC (2011) Liberal use of tricuspid-valve annuloplasty during left-ventricular assist device implantation. *Eur J Cardiothorac Surg* 41:213–217.

[7] Piacentino V, Williams ML, Depp T, Garcia-Huerta K, Blue L, Lodge AJ, Mackensen GB, Swaminathan M, Rogers JG, Milano CA (2011) Impact of Tricuspid Valve Regurgitation in Patients Treated With Implantable Left Ventricular Assist Devices. *Ann Thorac Surg* 91:1342–1347.

[8] Piacentino V, Troupes CD, Ganapathi AM, et al. (2011) Clinical Impact of Concomitant Tricuspid Valve Procedures During Left Ventricular Assist Device Implantation. *Ann Thorac Surg* 92:1414–1419.

[9] Saeed D, Kidambi T, Shalli S, Lapin B, Malaisrie SC, Lee R, Cotts WG, McGee EC (2011) Tricuspid valve repair with left ventricular assist device implantation: Is it warranted? *J Heart Lung Transplant* 30:530–535.

[10] Deo SV, Hasin T, Altarabsheh SE, McKellar SH, Shah IK, III LD, Stulak JM, Daly RC, Park SJ, Joyce LD (2012) Concomitant Tricuspid Valve Repair or Replacement During Left Ventricular Assist Device Implant Demonstrates Comparable Outcomes in the Long Term. *J Card Surg* 27:760–766.

[11] Maltais S, Topilsky Y, Tchantchaleishvili V, McKellar SH, Durham LA, Joyce LD, Daly RC, Park SJ (2012) Surgical treatment of tricuspid valve insufficiency promotes early reverse remodeling in

patients with axial-flow left ventricular assist devices. *J Thorac Cardiovasc Surg* 143:1370–1376.e1.

[12] Morgan JA, Tsiouris A, Nemeh HW, Hodari A, Karam J, Brewer RJ, Paone G (2013) Impact of concomitant cardiac procedures performed during implantation of long-term left ventricular assist devices. *J Heart Lung Transplant* 32:1255–1261.

[13] Akhter SA, Salabat MR, Philip JL, Valeroso TB, Russo MJ, Rich JD, Jeevanandam V (2014) Durability of De Vega Tricuspid Valve Annuloplasty for Severe Tricuspid Regurgitation During Left Ventricular Assist Device Implantation. *Ann Thorac Surg* 98:81–83.

[14] Brewer RJ, Cabrera R, El-Atrache M, et al. (2014) Relationship of Tricuspid Repair at the Time of Left Ventricular Assist Device Implantation and Survival. *Int J Artif Organs* 37:834–838.

[15] Fujita T, Kobayashi J, Hata H, Seguchi O, Murata Y, Yanase M, Nakatani T (2014) Right heart failure and benefits of adjuvant tricuspid valve repair in patients undergoing left ventricular assist device implantation. *Eur J Cardiothorac Surg* 46:802–807.

[16] John R, Naka Y, Park SJ, Sai-Sudhakar C, Salerno C, Sundareswaran KS, Farrar DJ, Milano CA (2014) Impact of concurrent surgical valve procedures in patients receiving continuous-flow devices. *J Thorac Cardiovasc Surg* 147:581–589.

[17] Robertson JO, Grau-Sepulveda MV, Okada S, O'Brien SM, Brennan JM, Shah AS, Itoh A, Damiano RJ, Prasad S, Silvestry SC (2014) Concomitant tricuspid valve surgery during implantation of continuous-flow left ventricular assist devices: A Society of Thoracic Surgeons database analysis. *J Heart Lung Transplant* 33:609–617.

[18] Oezpeker C, Zittermann A, Paluszkiewicz L, Piran M, Puehler T, Sayin AO, Ensminger S, Milting H, Morshuis M, Gummert JF (2015) Tricuspid valve repair in patients with left-ventricular assist device implants and tricuspid valve regurgitation: propensity score-adjusted analysis of clinical outcome. *Interact Cardiovasc Thorac Surg* 21:741–747.

[19] Goldraich L, Kawajiri H, Foroutan F, Braga J, Billia P, Misurka J, Stansfield WE, Yau T, Ross HJ, Rao V (2016) Tricuspid Valve

Annular Dilation as a Predictor of Right Ventricular Failure After Implantation of a Left Ventricular Assist Device. *J Card Surg* 31:110–116.

[20] Han J, Takeda K, Takayama H, et al. (2016) Durability and clinical impact of tricuspid valve procedures in patients receiving a continuous-flow left ventricular assist device. *J Thorac Cardiovasc Surg* 151:520–527.e1.

[21] Song HK, Gelow JM, Mudd J, Chien C, Tibayan FA, Hollifield K, Naftel D, Kirklin J (2016) Limited Utility of Tricuspid Valve Repair at the Time of Left Ventricular Assist Device Implantation. *Ann Thorac Surg* 101:2168–2174.

[22] Drakos SG, Janicki L, Horne BD, et al. (2010) Risk Factors Predictive of Right Ventricular Failure After Left Ventricular Assist Device Implantation. *Am J Cardiol* 105:1030–1035.

[23] Kormos RL, Teuteberg JJ, Pagani FD, et al. (2010) Right ventricular failure in patients with the HeartMate II continuous-flow left ventricular assist device: Incidence, risk factors, and effect on outcomes. *J Thorac Cardiovasc Surg* 139:1316–1324.

[24] Pinney SP (2012) The role of tricuspid valve repair and replacement in right heart failure. *Curr Opin Cardiol* 27:288–295.

[25] Antunes MJ, Rodríguez-Palomares J, Prendergast B, et al. (2017) Management of tricuspid valve regurgitation: Position statement of the European Society of Cardiology Working Groups of Cardiovascular Surgery and Valvular Heart Disease. *Eur J Cardiothorac Surg* 52:1022–1030.

[26] Neragi-Miandoab S, Goldstein D, Bello R, Michler R, D'Alessandro D (2012) Right ventricular dysfunction following continuous flow left ventriccular assist device placement in 51 patients: predicators and outcomes. *J Cardiothorac Surg.* doi: 10.1186/1749-8090-7-60.

[27] Dreyfus GD, Corbi PJ, Chan KMJ, Bahrami T (2005) Secondary tricuspid regurgitation or dilatation: which should be the criteria for surgical repair? *Ann Thorac Surg* 79:127–132.

[28] Taramasso M, Vanermen H, Maisano F, Guidotti A, La Canna G, Alfieri O (2012) The growing clinical importance of secondary tricuspid regurgitation. *J Am Coll Cardiol* 59:703–710.

[29] Kukucka M, Stepanenko A, Potapov E, Krabatsch T, Kuppe H, Habazettl H (2012) Impact of tricuspid valve annulus dilation on mid-term survival after implantation of a left ventricular assist device. *J Heart Lung Transplant* 31:967–971.

[30] Moon MR, Stinson EB, Miller DC (1997) Surgical treatment of endocarditis. *Prog Cardiovasc Dis* 40:239–264.

[31] Kavarana MN, Pessin-Minsley MS, Urtecho J, Catanese KA, Flannery M, Oz MC, Naka Y (2002) Right ventricular dysfunction and organ failure in left ventricular assist device recipients: a continuing problem. *Ann Thorac Surg* 73:745–750.

[32] Lee S, Kamdar F, Madlon-Kay R, Boyle A, Colvin-Adams M, Pritzker M, John R (2010) Effects of the HeartMate II continuous-flow left ventricular assist device on right ventricular function. *J Heart Lung Transplant* 29:209–215.

[33] Bellavia D, Iacovoni A, Scardulla C, et al. (2017) Prediction of right ventricular failure after ventricular assist device implant: systematic review and meta-analysis of observational studies. *Eur J Heart Fail* 19:926–946.

[34] Potapov EV, Stepanenko A, Dandel M, Kukucka M, Lehmkuhl HB, Weng Y, Hennig F, Krabatsch T, Hetzer R (2008) Tricuspid Incompetence and Geometry of the Right Ventricle as Predictors of Right Ventricular Function After Implantation of a Left Ventricular Assist Device. *J Heart Lung Transplant* 27:1275–1281.

[35] Jang JY, Heo R, Lee S, Kim JB, Kim D-H, Yun S-C, Song J-M, Song J-K, Lee J-W, Kang D-H (2017) Comparison of Results of Tricuspid Valve Repair Versus Replacement for Severe Functional Tricuspid Regurgitation. *Am J Cardiol* 119:905–910.

[36] McCarthy PM, Bhudia SK, Rajeswaran J, Hoercher KJ, Lytle BW, Cosgrove DM, Blackstone EH (2004) Tricuspid valve repair: durability and risk factors for failure. *J Thorac Cardiovasc Surg* 127:674–685.

[37] Belluschi I, Forno BD, Lapenna E, Nisi T, Iaci G, Ferrara D, Castiglioni A, Alfieri O, Bonis MD (2018) Surgical Techniques for Tricuspid Valve Disease. *Front Cardiovasc Med.* doi: 10.3389/fcvm.2018.00118.

[38] Taramasso M, Maisano F (2017) Transcatheter tricuspid valve intervention: state of the art. *EuroIntervention* 13:AA40–AA50.

[39] Krishnaswamy A, Navia J, Kapadia SR (2018) Transcatheter Tricuspid Valve Replacement. *Interv Cardiol Clin* 7:65–70.

[40] Taramasso M, Alessandrini H, Latib A, et al. (2019) Outcomes After Current Transcatheter Tricuspid Valve Intervention. *JACC Cardiovasc Interv* 12:155–165.

[41] Hahn RT, George I, Kodali SK, et al. (2019) Early Single-Site Experience With Transcatheter Tricuspid Valve Replacement. JACC Cardiovasc Imaging 12:416–429.

[42] Søndergaard L, Gustafsson F (2019) The Potential Role of Transcatheter Heart Valve Interventions in Heart Failure Treatment. *JACC Cardiovasc Interv* 12:166–168.

[43] Chan MCY, Giannetti N, Kato T, Kornbluth M, Oyer P, Valantine HA, Robbins RC, Hunt SA (2001) Severe tricuspid regurgitation after heart transplantation. *J Heart Lung Transplant* 20:709–717.

[44] Filsoufi F, Salzberg SP, Anderson CA, Couper GS, Cohn LH, Adams DH (2006) Optimal Surgical Management of Severe Tricuspid Regurgitation in Cardiac Transplant Patients. *J Heart Lung Transplant* 25:289–293.

[45] Berger Y, Zahav YH, Kassif Y, Kogan A, Kuperstein R, Freimark D, Lavee J (2012) Tricuspid Valve Regurgitation after Orthotopic Heart Transplantation: Prevalence and Etiology. *J Transplant* 2012:1–8.

[46] Herrmann G, Simon R, Haverich A, Cremer J, Dammenhayn L, Schafers H, Wahlers T, Borst H (1989) Left ventricular function, tricuspid incompetence, and incidence of coronary artery disease late after orthotopic heart transplantation. *Eur J Cardiothorac Surg* 3:111–118.

[47] Lewis MJ, Ginns JN, Ye S, Chai P, Quaegebeur JM, Bacha E, Rosenbaum MS (2016) Postoperative tricuspid regurgitation after

adult congenital heart surgery is associated with adverse clinical outcomes. *J Thorac Cardiovasc Surg* 151:460–465.
[48] Anderson CA, Shernan SK, Leacche M, et al. (2004) Severity of Intraoperative Tricuspid Regurgitation Predicts Poor Late Survival Following Cardiac Transplantation. *Ann Thorac Surg* 78:1635–1642.
[49] Brown NE, Muehlebach GF, Jones P, Gorton ME, Stuart RS, Borkon AM (2004) Tricuspid annuloplasty significantly reduces early tricuspid regurgitation after biatrial heart transplantation. *J Heart Lung Transplant* 23:1160–1162.
[50] Jeevanandam V, Russell H, Mather P, Furukawa S, Anderson A, Raman J (2006) Donor Tricuspid Annuloplasty During Orthotopic Heart Transplantation: Long-Term Results of a Prospective Controlled Study. *Ann Thorac Surg* 82:2089–2095.
[51] Sales VL, McCarthy PM (2010) Durability of Functional Tricuspid Valve Repair. *Semin Thorac Cardiovasc Surg* 22:97–103.
[52] Bishawi M, Zanotti G, Shaw L, et al. (2018) Tricuspid Valve Regurgitation Immediately After Heart Transplant and Long-Term Outcomes. *Ann Thorac Surg.* doi: 10.1016/j.athoracsur.2018.10.065.
[53] Greenberg J, Teman NR, Haft JW, Romano MA, Pagani FD, Aaronson KD, Wu AH (2018) Association of Donor Tricuspid Valve Repair With Outcomes After Cardiac Transplantation. *Ann Thorac Surg* 105:542–547.
[54] Badiwala MV, Rao V (2007) Tricuspid valve replacement after cardiac transplantation. *Curr Opin Cardiol* 22:123–127.
[55] Fiorelli AI, Stolf NAG, Filho CACA, Santos RHB, Buco FHA, Fiorelli LR, Issa V, Bacal F, Bocchi EA (2007) Prophylactic Donor Tricuspid Annuloplasty in Orthotopic Bicaval Heart Transplantation. *Transplant Pro*c 39:2527–2530.
[56] Bollano E, Karason K, Lidén H, Dellgren G (2016) How should we manage early tricuspid valve regurgitation after heart transplantation? *Int J Cardiol* 214:191–193.
[57] Yankah A (2000) Tricuspid valve dysfunction and surgery after orthotopic cardiac transplantation. *Eur J Cardiothorac Surg* 17:343–348.

[58] Topilsky Y, Khanna A, Le Toumeau T, Park S, Michelena H, Suri R, Mahoney DW, Enriquez-Sarano M (2012) Clinical context and mechanism of functional tricuspid regurgitation in patients with and without pulmonary hypertension. *Circ Cardiovasc Imaging* 5:314–323.

[59] Nguyen V, Cantarovich M, Cecere R, Giannetti N (2005) Tricuspid regurgitation after cardiac transplantation: how many biopsies are too many? *J Heart Lung Transplant Off Publ Int Soc Heart Transplant.* doi: 10.1016/j.healun.2004.07.007.

[60] Mielniczuk L, Haddad H, Davies RA, Veinot JP (2005) Tricuspid Valve Chordal Tissue in Endomyocardial Biopsy Specimens of Patients With Significant Tricuspid Regurgitation. *J Heart Lung Transplant* 24:1586–1590.

[61] Koch A, Remppis A, Dengler T, Schnabel P, Hagl S, Sack F (2005) Influence of different implantation techniques on AV valve competence after orthotopic heart transplantation. *Eur J Cardiothorac Surg* 28:717–723.

[62] Williams MJA, Lee M-Y, DiSalvo TG, Dec GW, Picard MH, Palacios IF, Semigran MJ (1996) Biopsy-induced flail tricuspid leaflet and tricuspid regurgitation following orthotopic cardiac transplantation. *Am J Cardiol* 77:1339–1344.

[63] Laske A, Carrel T, Niederhauser U, Pasic M, von Segesser L, Jenni R, Turina M (1995) Modified operation technique for orthotopic heart transplantation. *Eur J Cardiothorac Surg* 9:120–126.

[64] Aziz T, Burgess M, Khafagy R, Hann AW, Campbell C, Rahman A, Deiraniya A, Yonan N (1999) Bicaval and standard techniques in orthotopic heart transplantation: Medium-term experience in cardiac performance and survival. *J Thorac Cardiovasc Surg* 118:115–122.

[65] Jacob S, Sellke F (2009) Is bicaval orthotopic heart transplantation superior to the biatrial technique? *Interact Cardiovasc Thorac Surg* 9:333–342.

[66] Marelli D, Silvestry SC, Zwas D, Mather P, Rubin S, Dempsey AF, Stein L, Rodriguez E, Diehl JT, Feldman AM (2007) Modified

inferior vena caval anastomosis to reduce tricuspid valve regurgitation after heart transplantation. *Tex Heart Inst J* 34:30–35.

[67] Davies RR, Russo MJ, Morgan JA, Sorabella RA, Naka Y, Chen JM (2010) Standard versus bicaval techniques for orthotopic heart transplantation: An analysis of the United Network for Organ Sharing database. *J Thorac Cardiovasc Surg* 140:700–708.e2.

[68] Lund LH, Edwards LB, Kucheryavaya AY, et al. (2013) The Registry of the International Society for Heart and Lung Transplantation: Thirtieth Official Adult Heart Transplant Report—2013$\mathsemicolon$ Focus Theme: Age. *J Heart Lung Transplant* 32:951–964.

[69] Kobashigawa J, Patel J, Azarbal B, et al. (2015) Randomized Pilot Trial of Gene Expression Profiling Versus Heart Biopsy in the First Year After Heart Transplant. *Circ Heart Fail* 8:557–564.

[70] Yusen RD, Edwards LB, Dipchand AI, Goldfarb SB, Kucheryavaya AY, Levvey BJ, Lund LH, Meiser B, Rossano JW, Stehlik J (2016) The Registry of the International Society for Heart and Lung Transplantation: Thirty-third Adult Lung and Heart–Lung Transplant Report—2016$\mathsemicolon$ Focus Theme: Primary Diagnostic Indications for Transplant. *J Heart Lung Transplant* 35:1170–1184.

[71] Crumbley AJ, Bakel ABV (1994) Tricuspid valve repair for biopsy-induced regurgitation after cardiac transplantation. *Ann Thorac Surg* 58:1156–1160.

[72] Fiorelli AI, Coelho GHB, Aiello VD, Benvenuti LA, Palazzo JF, Júnior VPS, Canizares B, Dias RR, Stolf NAG (2012) Tricuspid Valve Injury After Heart Transplantation Due to Endomyocardial Biopsy: An Analysis of 3550 Biopsies. *Transplant Proc* 44:2479–2482.

[73] Alfieri O, Bonis MD, Lapenna E, Agricola E, Quarti A, Maisano F (2003) The "clover technique" as a novel approach for correction of post-traumatic tricuspid regurgitation. *J Thorac Cardiovasc Surg* 126:75–79.

[74] Fayad G, Modine T, Ennezat P-V, et al. (2005) The "clover technique" as a new approach for correction of postendocarditic

severe tricuspid valve regurgitation. *J Thorac Cardiovasc Surg* 130:1208–1210.

[75] Pozzi M, Pavlakovic I, Dondas A, Sebbag L, Boissonnat P, Obadia JF (2016) The clover technique in endomyocardial biopsy-induced tricuspid regurgitation. *Int J Cardiol* 203:731–732.

[76] Lapenna E, Bonis MD, Verzini A, Canna GL, Ferrara D, Calabrese MC, Taramasso M, Alfieri O (2010) The clover technique for the treatment of complex tricuspid valve insufficiency: midterm clinical and echocardiographic results in 66 patients. *Eur J Cardiothorac Surg* 37:1297–1303.

[77] Alhareti R, Bader F, Kfoury A, Hammond M, Karwande S, Gilbert E, Doty D, Hagan M, Thomas H, Renlund ta (2006) Tricuspid Valve Replacement After Cardiac Transplantation. *J Heart Lung Transplant* 25:48–52.

[78] Raghavan R, Cecere R, Cantarovich M, Giannetti N (2006) Tricuspid valve replacement after cardiac transplantation. *Clin Transplant* 20:673–676.

[79] Hafiz AM, Shih J, Kakouros N (2017) Transcatheter Tricuspid Valve Replacement in Orthotopic Heart Transplant. *J Invasive Cardiol* 29:E75–E76.

In: The Rediscovered Tricuspid Valve
Editor: Giacomo Bianchi
ISBN: 978-1-53616-098-7

Chapter 12

SURGICAL TREATMENT OF FUNCTIONAL TRICUSPID VALVE DISEASE: SURGEON'S PERSPECTIVE – INDICATIONS, RISK STRATIFICATION AND OUTCOMES

Giacomo Bianchi, MD, PhD,
Rafik Margaryan, MD, PhD and Marco Solinas*, MD
Department of Adult Cardiac Surgery, Ospedale del Cuore,
Fondazione Toscana "G. Monasterio," Massa, Italy

ABSTRACT

Surgery remains the gold-standard treatment of tricuspid insufficiency to date. Some misconceptions have systematically denied the importance of the surgical treatment of this valve, leading to an increase in long-term sequelae; these consequences are reflected in the presence of patients at higher risk who often make this type of treatment impossible due to the high risk. Accurate stratification of patients with primary or more often functional tricuspid valve disease is critical to

* Corresponding Author Email: marco.solinas@ftgm.it.

selecting who may benefit from surgery. Nevertheless, surgical techniques also play a key role, as they have an impact on the short- and long-term prognosis and must be adopted depending on the pathophysiological mechanism that determines tricuspid insufficiency. In this way, by selecting the right patient at the right time, operated with the right technique, results can be improved.

Keywords: risk stratification, functional tricuspid valve disease, surgical management

INTRODUCTION

Surgery is currently considered the gold-standard treatment of tricuspid insufficiency, while drug management is a palliative alternative.

The problems that the surgeon faces in defining the therapeutic path of the patient suffering from tricuspid valve insufficiency are essentially three:

1. persistence of the historical concept, in certain areas crystallized despite the evidence, that functional tricuspid insufficiency regresses almost invariably after correction of left heart disease (LHD) and that, if persistent, it is a pathology with a benign and indolent course;
2. the lack of a clear stratification of individual risk in isolated tricuspid pathology; in particular, the lack of a clear definition of advanced or non-reversible right ventricular dysfunction:
3. lack of clear indications for treatment in non-severe tricuspid valve insufficiency associated with LHD and which indicators to consider, as well as accesses and surgical techniques to be adopted and their impact on the prognosis.

In this chapter we will illustrate the past and current evidence that can help the surgeon in the peri-operative management of the patient with tricuspid insufficiency.

"FUNCTIONAL" TRICUSPID REGURGITATION IS NOT A SELF-LIMITING OR BENIGN DISEASE

The term "functional" insufficiency associated with tricuspid valve regurgitation secondary to LHD was coined in 1950 in a historical study about the venous pulse in this disease. This implies the idea that such valve regurgitation could resolve after correction of LHD [1].

In his 1967 study, Braunwald et al. analyzed the clinical and hemodynamic data of 28 patients with mitral pathology associated with severe tricuspid insufficiency who underwent cardiac surgery. All patients had a mitral valve replacement, while only 3 patients had a concomitant tricuspid annuloplasty. From the results of cardiac catheterization after surgery and the ability of patients to remain symptom-free at follow-up, the authors concluded that most patients had a reduction or resolution of tricuspid regurgitation after mitral correction; associated tricuspid surgery was therefore not indicated [2].

This vision has remained predominant in clinical practice for at least two decades. On the contrary, already in the first half of the 1970s, Carpentier et al. proposed the routine application of tricuspid repair in patients with functional pathology [3].

The consequences of this therapeutic approach became evident after the wider application of cardiac surgery due to technological improvements and better results in terms of peri-operative mortality. Since the late 1970s, many physicians have observed the development of heart failure in the long-term survivor patients as a result of severe tricuspid insufficiency [4, 5]; the operative mortality was high and the outcomes very poor in this subset of patients, so much so that some investigators began to call for a more liberal approach to tricuspid valve annuloplasty at the time of mitral valve surgery [6, 7].

The more recent report that severe TR resolved in more than 70% of patients undergoing pulmonary thromboendarterectomy, further propagated the misconception of fTR as a reversible and fairly benign disease [8].

The fate of untreated functional tricuspid insufficiency has been well outlined by studies of mitral balloon valvotomy, since the chest remains closed and the TV is left untreated.

Between 49% and 80% of patients with concomitant moderate or severe fTR did not experience a reduction in tricuspid valve insufficiency despite successful balloon valvotomy [9, 10]. Factors that emerge as most involved in fTR persistence are advanced age, pulmonary hypertension that does not resolve in the first days or weeks post-valvotomy and the presence of atrial fibrillation.

In a comparative study between balloon valvotomy and mitral surgery with prosthetic replacement in patients with concomitant severe tricuspid insufficiency, in the AF subgroup who had undergone surgery, event-free survival at 7 years was significantly better than in those who had received valvotomy alone; moreover, more than 92% of patients in the surgical arm were free from TR ≥ 2+/4+, compared to 46% in the valvotomy group [11].

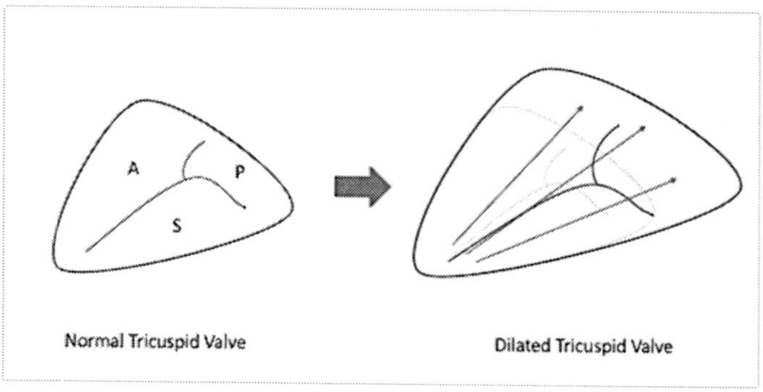

Figure 1. Tricuspid Valve dilatation represented schematically. The effect of right atrial enlargment along with leaflet tethering lead to annular dilatation towards the antero-posterior commisure (arrows). A: anterior leaflet; P: posterior leaflet; S: septal leaflet.

From a pathophysiological point of view, we can say that the increase in the size of the left atrium and of the pressures can trigger atrial fibrillation, which determines a dilation of the tricuspid annulus, hence the functional insufficiency; therefore, more the size of the right atrium and the atrial fibrillation contribute to the determinism of the annular dilatation than other forces such as the right ventricular remodeling (Figure 1).

In the case of pulmonary hypertension, its occurrence or failure to regress after valvotomy or surgery is due to a series of pathophysiological mechanisms; its immediate regression is often determined by the elimination of the passive component (post-capillary) and is influenced by the degree of decrease in left atrial pressure, residual mitral stenosis or the degree of mitral valve regurgitation; moreover, a progressive reduction in pulmonary hypertension occurs in young subjects by resolution of the vasoreactive component. This is in line with what has been reported in the literature, i.e., that pre-operative pulmonary hypertension does not correlate with late fTR [12].

In particular, one study shows that patients with high pre-operative pulmonary pressure (78 ± 14 mmHg vs 41 ± 6 mmHg) and moderate TR associated with mitral stenosis, have a degree of tricuspid insufficiency lower than follow-up than the other group [13]. The most reliable explanation is that patients with non-severe pulmonary hypertension had worse right ventricular function. This observation leads us directly to the second problem we are dealing with.

Risk Stratification in Functional Tricuspid Regurgitation. Role of Right Ventricular Function Assessment

Even after decades of a modern approach to tricuspid valve disease, the clinical identification of a tricuspid regurgitation that may represent a significant impact on the patient's clinic remains a challenge. Most clinical manifestations are determined by the underlying LHD [14], while symptoms of right heart disease are usually present in advanced stages and to be correlated with a reduction of cardiac output (fatigue) or systemic congestion (jugular pulsatility, hepatomegaly, splenomegaly, peripheral edema and ascites). The tricuspid murmur, at the left parasternal edge, has a marked inspiratory accentuation, but it can also be absent in the case of massive regurgitation.

From a laboratory point of view, congestive hepatopathy, besides being often asymptomatic, presents with alteration of the liver function indexes of cholestatic type (increase of Alkaline Phosphatase, gamma-glutamyl-transferase and serum bilirubin), rather than hepatic. It is also associated with reduced protein synthesis with hypoalbuminemia.

Renal dysfunction may also be present and its connection with tricuspid valve insufficiency is well established: the increase in central venous pressure with retrograde repercussion alters post-glomerular and post-capillary pressures, leading to parenchymal hypoperfusion and reduction of the filtrate. Further, not only the presence of tricuspid valve insufficiency with preserved right ventricular function can lead to this eventuality, but especially the concomitant dysfunction of the right ventricle is associated with increased mortality [15].

Further, hypersplenism may cause a reduction in haemoglobin levels; a preparatory cut-off of 11.3 g/dL has been suggested as a threshold value in identifying patients with event-free survival in isolated post-surgical fTR [16]. Finally, a level of BNP ≥200 pg/ml was found to be associated with reduced survival in isolated forms [17].

Perioperative risk assessment is essential in cardiac surgery and particularly when considering the possibility of operating on a patient with advanced tricuspid pathology. Currently, there are two systems for calculating surgical risk, EuroSCORE II and STS score, derived respectively from the European and American databases [18, 19]. Very recently, the scoring system specifically developed by LaPar on the basis of the STS database has identified some variables associated with the outcome of patients operated by fTR; the analysis lacks an internal validation between the predicted and actual outcome and also does not consider the presence of liver failure or right ventricular function [20]. The Model for End-Stage Liver Disease (MELD) score in its extended version (INR, total bilirubin and creatinine) or simplified version (total bilirubin and creatinine) can be a valid tool to integrate the risk arising from liver impairment of tricuspid disease [21, 22].

As you can see, there is still an elusive characterization of the right ventricle in tricuspid pathology.

The current North American and European guidelines of the Society for Echocardiography identify tricuspid regurgitation in three stages based on qualitative, semi-quantitative and quantitative parameters [23, 24]; in order to reduce intraobserver variability and increase diagnostic accuracy, a new algorithm has been proposed [25].

If we focus on the evaluation of the right ventricle, not a single value currently represents the gold-standard nor correlates with the outcome; the surgeon must rely on the integration of several factors. In the forms of fTR, ventricular magnification is the cause of valvular insufficiency; from an initial tethering of the leaflets we move on to annular dilatation which, by increasing the degree of regurgitation, produces further ventricular dilatation. The right ventricular enlargement resulting from septal dysfunction that can occur dyskinetic or akinetic produces a tethering of the septal leaflet causing insufficiency and perpetuating the vicious circle; the myocardial septal shift in turn compromises the left ventricular function and this has a negative impact on the stroke volume of the right ventricle [26, 27].

In clinical practice, the simplest method of assessing right ventricular dilation is to measure the end-systolic area edge and linear dimensions in end-diastole. At basal diameter >42 mm, mid cavity diameter >33 mm and apex-to-base length >86 mm indicate RV enlargement [28]; the same authors propose a FAC <35% and RV dP/dT <400 mmHg/sec as criteria for RV dysfunction beyond anatomic measures.

The ESC guidelines identify in a TAPSE <15 mm, TASV <11 cm/sec and RV ES area >20 cm2 the useful values in defining patients with RV dysfunction [29].

In part these values are taken from Lange et al. specifically the FAC <35%, a RIMP > 0.43 (pulsed doppler) or >0.54 (tissue doppler), S' < 9.5 cm/sec, global longitudinal free wall strain -20% (or absolute value <20%), while there is no agreement on the cut-off value of the TAPSE, which they referred to as <17 mm [30].

The use of right catheterization in selected patients may accurately indicate pulmonary pressures, vascular resistance and reversibility as well as the ability of the right ventricle to generate pressure, which is particularly important in view of the surgical reduction of the degree of valvular insufficiency [31].

With regard to the use of magnetic resonance imaging and CT scanning in the evaluation of the right ventricle, see the extensive discussion in the relevant chapter of this book.

It emerges, therefore, from the evidences exposed up to now regarding the stratification of the risk and the evaluation of the right ventricle in the fTR, how much more the decision to operate is based on parameters that must be integrated and how much more it is necessary from a research point of view to reach an integrated vision of when to intervene or when to manage in a medical way the right tricuspid regurgitation and advanced ventricular dysfunction.

Surgical Management of Tricuspid Valve Disease. Primary TR and Focus on Functional and Isolated Valve Disease

The surgical treatment of tricuspid insufficiency, although it represents the only definitive cure, is still today the subject of heated debate and discussion. This controversy is the consequence of the heterogeneity of the pathology (primary, functional, isolated forms) and the lack of solid evidence, especially in borderline cases or those not covered by the guidelines.

The European and North American guidelines are reported in comparison with the respective levels of evidence in the individual recommendations in Table 1.

Table 1. European and North American guidelines for surgical treatment of Tricuspid Regurgitation. *AHA/ACC 2014 guidelines (Nishimura et al. J Am Coll Cardiol 63, e57-e185 - 2014); **ESC/EACTS 2017 guidelines

	Level of Evidence and Class of Recommendation	
Primary tricuspid regurgitation	AHA/ACC (2014)*	ESC/EACTS (2017)**
Patients with severe primary tricuspid regurgitation undergoing left-sided valve surgery	I-C	I-C
Symptomatic severe isolated primary tricuspid regurgitation without severe right ventricular dysfunction	IIa-C	I-C
Patients with moderate primary tricuspid regurgitation undergoing left- sided valve surgery	-	IIa-C
Asymptomatic or mildly symptomatic severe isolated tricuspid regurgitation and progressive right ventricular dilatation or dysfunction	IIb-C	IIa-C
Secondary tricuspid regurgitation		
Patients with severe FTR undergoing left- sided valve surgery	I-C	I-C
Patients with mild or moderate FTR with a dilated annulus (≥40 mm or >21 mm/m2) undergoing left- sided valve surgery	IIa-B	IIa-C
Patients with mild or moderate FTR undergoing left- sided valve surgery even in the absence of annular dilatation when previous right heart failure has been documented	IIa-B	IIb-C
Patients with moderate FTR and pulmonary hypertension at the time of left- sided valve surgery	IIb-C	-
After previous left- sided surgery and in the absence of recurrent left- sided valve dysfunction, surgery should be considered in patients with severe FTR who are symptomatic or have progressive right ventricular dilatation or dysfunction, in the absence of severe right ventricular or left ventricular dysfunction and severe pulmonary vascular disease and/or hypertension	IIb-C	IIa-C

Baumgartner et al. *Eur Heart J* 38;36, 2739-2791 - 2017

Primary Tricuspid Regurgitation

Severe tricuspid insufficiency concomitant with left-sided heart disease surgery should be surgically treated at the same time. In the case of isolated severe disease, surgery is indicated if the patient remains symptomatic despite optimal medical treatment. Finally, treatment should be reserved for patients with severe insufficiency if asymptomatic or paucisymptomatic in the presence of a progressive dysfunction of the right ventricle but without a severe impairment of it, which would be a strong contraindication.

From an operating point of view, the surgery can be performed by a standard approach (median sternotomy) or by a minimally invasive approach, such as right lateral mini-thoracotomy [32]. The use of extracorporeal circulation is mandatory, although the surgery can be conducted without surviving the aorta and therefore at the beating heart.

In primary forms, reparability depends on the organic lesions; although success rates of up to 70% are reported, in some cases with complex anatomy or structural subversion, valve replacement is often preferred [33–35] (Figure 2); in some cases of endocarditis on refractory and extended tricuspid or where the risk of re-infection is high, valvulectomy is contemplated, postponing prosthetic replacement if the clinical scenario changes [36, 37].

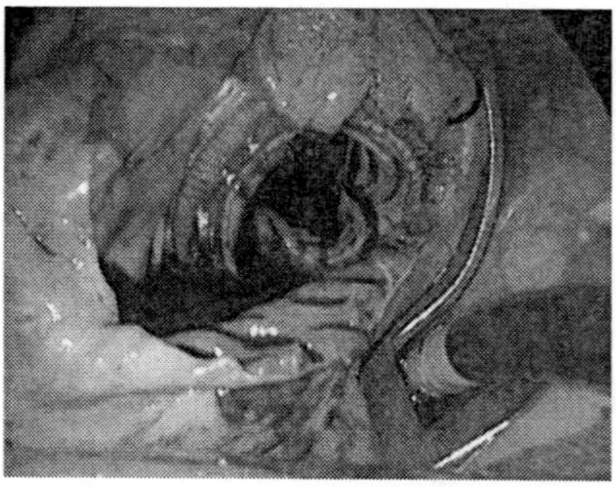

Figure 2. Tricuspid Valve Replacement. Note the opened right atrium and the bioprosthesis already in place (Photo courtesy of the Author (G. Bianchi), personal archive).

Functional TR at the Time of Left-Sided Heart Valve Surgery

The fundamental cornerstones of the surgical management of secondary insufficiency are the elimination of the right ventricle post-cardiac and the reduction of the size of the tricuspid annulus. The first point is implemented by the correction of left-heart disease and the optimization of left ventricular function, while the second point is made by a reductive annuloplasty of the valve [38].

Annular dilatation is constantly associated with tricuspid insufficiency; in some studies it is indicated that, in the case of an associated procedure, an annuloplasty must be performed if the annulus is dilated, regardless of the degree of valve regurgitation; in fact, it has been demonstrated by numerous studies that even moderate tricuspid insufficiency has a negative impact on the prognosis, especially when the annulus is enlarged [39–41].

According to the guidelines, action should be taken if a annulus is > 40 mm or > 21 mm/m^2 measured in four chambers at the echocardiogram or if there is a history of right ventricular failure [42, 43]. In addition, an intraoperative method was proposed by Dreyfus et al. to evaluate patients who should receive tricuspid surgery; the method involved measuring the distance between antero-septal commissure and antero-posterior commissure in diastolic arrest; if this measure was >70 mm, a restrictive annuloplasty was performed [44]. In our opinion, this method, quite obsolete, should not be the clinical trigger for intervention since it limits its applicability for patients operated on median sternotomy and would miss a significant proportion of patients that may benefit for tricuspid annuloplasty.

The addition of reparative tricuspid surgery to mitral surgery has proven particularly effective for the patient. A large study of 645 patients showed that concomitant and prophylactic repair of the tricuspid valve does not increase the risk of procedural and peri-procedural complications, primarily the risk of atrioventricular block and permanent pacemaker implantation; moreover, the benefits were long-lasting, in fact at 7 years of follow-up the degree of tricuspid insufficiency was lower and the right ventricular function better than those in whom it had not been treated [45].

Some reports, which consider a unified multi-center analysis, often national registers, indicate higher mortality in associated mitro-tricuspid procedures, with ranges between 8.5% and 11.7% [46, 47]. Although they are high, it must be remembered that they consider the cases in their entirety and in these, there are certainly patients with advanced dysfunction of the right ventricle; it is no coincidence that this prognosis is similar to the contemporary outcomes of isolated tricuspid surgery [48].

Isolated Functional Tricuspid Regurgitation

Although isolated tricuspid surgery is technically feasible in most patients, it is subject to high morbidity and mortality due to the presence of right ventricular dysfunction or chronic pulmonary disease [49]. In particular, isolated tricuspid insufficiency after LHD surgery is a clinical and surgical challenge; it is necessary to state that the 13% overall isolated TR surgery reported by a North American registry is largely underestimated, as a significant proportion of patients are not proposed for surgery because of advanced age, comorbidity or poor functional status [48]. Once again, careful selection of patients for concomitant or isolated tricuspid valve surgery requires a careful risk stratification and assessment of the right ventricle, as it is the main determinant of these patients' early and late outcome.

Surgical Treatment for Functional Tricuspid Regurgitation

The most commonly used technique for the surgical correction of tricuspid insufficiency is annuloplasty. It aims to reduce annular dilatation, restore valve geometry and lead to improved co-optation between the leaflets.

Two methods are used to perform it, one by suturing, the other by positioning a prosthetic ring. The suture method, proposed by De Vega, provides for a double suture line along the annulus except at the point where there is the projection of the atrio-ventricular node and the perforating portion of the His bundle [50]; its modifications provide for the regular interposition of pledgets to avoid the guitar string insufficiency that develops over time [51–53].

Implantation of a prosthetic ring blocks the valve in a systolic position [3] (Figure 3); many long-term studies have shown that the use of a prosthetic ring for repair is associated with a longer duration of the repair itself and confers an improvement in survival and freedom from events; in some series, in fact, freedom from moderate or severe TR is >85% in treatments with a prosthetic ring [54, 55].

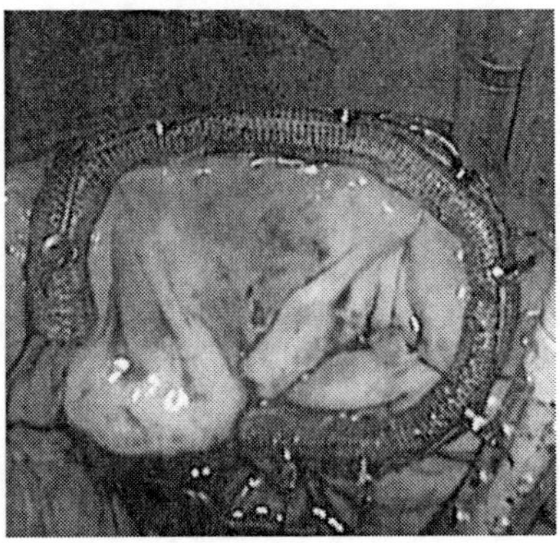

Figure 3. Tricuspid valve annuloplasty performed through endoscopic non-rib spreading right lateral mini-thoracotomy; Incomplete 3D ring is used. Note how annuloplasty blocks the valve in systole and the preponderance of the anterior leaflet (photo courtesy of the G. Bianchi, personal archive).

The first prosthetic rings used were bidimensional, while it is known that the tricuspid valve has a peculiar three-dimensional geometry [56]. Although the semi-rigid ring demonstrated very high freedom from re-intervention (97.5% at 10 years) [54], it has been suggested that the lack of respect for the three dimensions is associated with a failure of the valve repair [57]. Navia et al. compared the results of a two-dimensional ring with a prosthetic ring with a three-dimensional design, finding a moderate or severe TR recurrence incidence of 10% and 14% respectively at 5 years [58]. This incidence was also reported by another series of patients [59]; in particular, these investigators pointed out that in those who experienced such a recurrence of failure, the most important predictors were the degree of leaflet tethering and the presence of residual post-operative TV regurgitation.

In these cases it is necessary to use additional techniques; one of them is known as "Clover" technique, which consists in the suturing of the three margins of the valve leaflets associated with a annuloplasty with ring [60], with excellent results at follow-up [61].

Another technique is the so-called "augmentation" of the anterior leaflet in order to increase the co-optation surface and bring it back to the annular plane in case of important tethering, i.e., a coaptation height >8 mm; the peculiarity and effectiveness of this technique lies in the different geometry of the right outflow, so that even if redundant, the anterior tricuspid leaflet with patch will never be in contrast and sucked into the right outflow causing an obstruction [62]. Although very interesting as a concept, reproducibility may be poor and our group has proposed a technique for measuring and shaping the autologous pericardial patch [63].

Conclusion

Tricuspid valve failure is a major challenge for both the clinician and the surgeon. It requires an important integration between clinical-anamnestic data, general risk stratification and in particular an evaluation of the right ventricle.

Now that the concept of tricuspid insufficiency as a benign and self-limiting disease has been overcome, it is necessary to rely on multidisciplinary indices to identify which patients have been treated and how.

In the most frequent functional form, as well as in the primitive forms, a concomitant surgery of the tricuspid valve does not increase the risk of surgery, provided that the patient is carefully selected, producing a short and long-term improvement of the prognosis provided that the surgeon uses the right techniques, guided by knowledge of the mechanism of disease.

REFERENCES

[1] Messer AL, Hurst JW (1950) A study of the venous pulse in tricuspid valve disease. *Circulation* 1:388–393.

[2] Braunwald NS, Ross JR J, Morrow AG (1967) Conservative management of tricuspid regurgitation in patients undergoing mitral valve replacement. *Circulation* 35:I–63.

[3] Carpentier A, Deloche A, Hanania G, Forman J, Sellier P, Piwnica A, Dubost C, McGoon DC (1974) Surgical management of acquired tricuspid valve disease. *J Thorac Cardiovasc Surg* 67:53–65.

[4] Breyer RH, McClenathan JH, Michaelis LL, McIntosh CL, Morrow AG (1976) Tricuspid regurgitation. A comparison of nonoperative management, tricuspid annuloplasty, and tricuspid valve replacement. *J Thorac Cardiovasc Surg* 72:867–874.

[5] Simon R, Oelert H, Borst HG, Lichtlen PR (1980) Influence of mitral valve surgery on tricuspid incompetence concomitant with mitral valve disease. *Circulation* 62:I152-157.

[6] King RM, Schaff HV, Danielson GK, Gersh BJ, Orszulak TA, Piehler JM, Puga FJ, Pluth JR (1984) Surgery for tricuspid regurgitation late after mitral valve replacement. *Circulation* 70:I193–7.

[7] Groves PH, Hall RJ (1992) Late tricuspid regurgitation following mitral valve surgery. *J Heart Valve Dis* 1:80–86.

[8] Sadeghi HM, Kimura BJ, Raisinghani A, Blanchard DG, Mahmud E, Fedullo PF, Jamieson SW, DeMaria AN (2004) Does lowering pulmonary arterial pressure eliminate severe functional tricuspid regurgitation? Insights from pulmonary thromboendarterectomy. *J Am Coll Cardiol* 44:126–132.

[9] Sagie A, Schwammenthal E, Palacios IF, King ME, Leavitt M, Freitas N, Weyman AE, Levine RA (1994) Significant tricuspid regurgitation does not resolve after percutaneous balloon mitral valvotomy. *J Thorac Cardiovasc Surg* 108:727–735.

[10] Hannoush H, Fawzy ME, Stefadouros M, Moursi M, Chaudhary MA, Dunn B (2004) Regression of significant tricuspid regurgitation after

mitral balloon valvotomy for severe mitral stenosis. *Am Heart J* 148:865–870.

[11] Song J-M, Kim S-D, Kim J-H, Kim M-J, Kang D-H, Seo JB, Lim T-H, Lee JW, Song M-G, Song J-K (2007) Long-term predictors of descending aorta aneurysmal change in patients with aortic dissection. *J Am Coll Cardiol* 50:799–804.

[12] Porter A, Shapira Y, Wurzel M, Sulkes J, Vaturi M, Adler Y, Sahar G, Sagie A (1999) Tricuspid regurgitation late after mitral valve replacement: clinical and echocardiographic evaluation. *J Heart Valve Dis* 8:57–62.

[13] Kaul TK, Ramsdale DR, Mercer JL (1991) Functional tricuspid regurgitation following replacement of the mitral valve. *Int J Cardiol* 33:305–313.

[14] Rodés-Cabau J, Taramasso M, O'Gara PT (2016) Diagnosis and treatment of tricuspid valve disease: current and future perspectives. *The Lancet* 388:2431–2442.

[15] Agricola E, Marini C, Stella S, et al. (2017) Effects of functional tricuspid regurgitation on renal function and long-term prognosis in patients with heart failure. *J Cardiovasc Med Hagerstown Md* 18:60–68.

[16] Kim H-K, Kim Y-J, Park J-S, Kim KH, Kim K-B, Ahn H, Sohn D-W, Oh B-H, Park Y-B, Choi Y-S (2006) Determinants of the Severity of Functional Tricuspid Regurgitation. *Am J Cardiol* 98:236–242.

[17] Yoon C-H, Zo J-H, Kim Y-J, et al. (2010) B-type natriuretic Peptide in isolated severe tricuspid regurgitation: determinants and impact on outcome. *J Cardiovasc Ultrasound* 18:139–145.

[18] Nashef SAM, Roques F, Sharples LD, Nilsson J, Smith C, Goldstone AR, Lockowandt U (2012) EuroSCORE II. *Eur J Cardio-Thorac Surg Off J Eur Assoc Cardio-Thorac Surg* 41:734–744; discussion 744-745.

[19] O'Brien SM, Shahian DM, Filardo G, et al. (2009) The Society of Thoracic Surgeons 2008 cardiac surgery risk models: part 2--isolated valve surgery. *Ann Thorac Surg* 88:S23-42.

[20] LaPar DJ, Likosky DS, Zhang M, et al. (2018) Development of a Risk Prediction Model and Clinical Risk Score for Isolated Tricuspid Valve Surgery. *Ann Thorac Surg* 106:129–136.

[21] Ailawadi G, Lapar DJ, Swenson BR, Siefert SA, Lau C, Kern JA, Peeler BB, Littlewood KE, Kron IL (2009) Model for end-stage liver disease predicts mortality for tricuspid valve surgery. *Ann Thorac Surg* 87:1460–1467; discussion 1467-1468.

[22] Tsuda K, Koide M, Kunii Y, Watanabe K, Miyairi S, Ohashi Y, Harada T (2013) Simplified model for end-stage liver disease score predicts mortality for tricuspid valve surgery. *Interact Cardiovasc Thorac Surg* 16:630–635.

[23] Zoghbi WA, Adams D, Bonow RO, et al. (2017) Recommendations for Noninvasive Evaluation of Native Valvular Regurgitation. *J Am Soc Echocardiogr* 30:303–371.

[24] Lancellotti P, Tribouilloy C, Hagendorff A, Popescu BA, Edvardsen T, Pierard LA, Badano L, and JLZ (2013) Recommendations for the echocardiographic assessment of native valvular regurgitation: an executive summary from the European Association of Cardiovascular Imaging. *Eur Heart J - Cardiovasc Imaging* 14:611–644.

[25] Grant ADM, Thavendiranathan P, Rodriguez LL, Kwon D, Marwick TH (2014) Development of a consensus algorithm to improve interobserver agreement and accuracy in the determination of tricuspid regurgitation severity. *J Am Soc Echocardiogr Off Publ Am Soc Echocardiogr* 27:277–284.

[26] Hoffman D, Sisto D, Frater RW, Nikolic SD (1994) Left-to-right ventricular interaction with a noncontracting right ventricle. *J Thorac Cardiovasc Surg* 107:1496–1502.

[27] Haddad F, Doyle R, Murphy DJ, Hunt SA (2008) Right ventricular function in cardiovascular disease, part II: Pathophysiology, clinical importance, and management of right ventricular failure. *Circulation* 117:1717–1731.

[28] Rudski LG, Lai WW, Afilalo J, Hua L, Handschumacher MD, Chandrasekaran K, Solomon SD, Louie EK, Schiller NB (2010) Guidelines for the echocardiographic assessment of the right heart in

adults: a report from the American Society of Echocardiography endorsed by the European Association of Echocardiography, a registered branch of the European Society of Cardiology, and the Canadian Society of Echocardiography. *J Am Soc Echocardiogr Off Publ Am Soc Echocardiogr* 23:685–713; quiz 786–788.

[29] Vahanian A PJ Pierard L, Dion R (2009) Valvular heart disease. In: *ESC Textb. Cardiovasc. Med.* Oxford University Press, pp 763–817.

[30] Lang RM, Badano LP, Mor-Avi V, et al. (2015) Recommendations for cardiac chamber quantification by echocardiography in adults: an update from the American Society of Echocardiography and the European Association of Cardiovascular Imaging. *J Am Soc Echocardiogr Off Publ Am Soc Echocardiogr* 28:1-39.e14.

[31] Rao S, Tate DA, Stouffer GA (2013) Hemodynamic findings in severe tricuspid regurgitation. *Catheter Cardiovasc Interv Off J Soc Card Angiogr Interv* 81:162–169.

[32] Urbandt P, Santana O, Mihos CG, Pineda AM, Joseph Lamelas null (2014) Minimally invasive approach for isolated tricuspid valve surgery. *J Heart Valve Dis* 23:783–787.

[33] Seeburger J, Borger MA, Passage J, Misfeld M, Holzhey D, Noack T, Sauer M, Ender J, Mohr FW (2010) Minimally invasive isolated tricuspid valve surgery. *J Heart Valve Dis* 19:189–192; discussion 193.

[34] Bevan PJW, Haydock DA, Kang N (2014) Long-term survival after isolated tricuspid valve replacement. *Heart Lung Circ* 23:697–702.

[35] De Meester P, Van De Bruaene A, Voigt J-U, Herijgers P, Budts W (2014) Outcome and determinants of prognosis in patients undergoing isolated tricuspid valve surgery: retrospective single center analysis. *Int J Cardiol* 175:333–339.

[36] Arbulu A, Holmes RJ, Asfaw I (1991) Tricuspid valvulectomy without replacement. Twenty years' experience. *J Thorac Cardiovasc* Surg 102:917–922.

[37] Miró JM, Moreno A, Mestres CA (2003) Infective Endocarditis in Intravenous Drug Abusers. *Curr Infect Dis Rep* 5:307–316.

[38] Raja SG, Dreyfus GD (2010) Basis for intervention on functional tricuspid regurgitation. *Semin Thorac Cardiovasc Surg* 22:79–83.

[39] Nath J, Foster E, Heidenreich PA (2004) Impact of Tricuspid Regurgitation on Long-Term Survival. *J Am Coll Cardiol* 43:405–409.

[40] Di Mauro M, Bivona A, Iacò AL, Contini M, Gagliardi M, Varone E, Gallina S, Calafiore AM (2009) Mitral valve surgery for functional mitral regurgitation: prognostic role of tricuspid regurgitation. *Eur J Cardio-Thorac Surg Off J Eur Assoc Cardio-Thorac Surg* 35:635–639; discussion 639-640.

[41] Van de Veire NR, Braun J, Delgado V, Versteegh MIM, Dion RA, Klautz RJM, Bax JJ (2011) Tricuspid annuloplasty prevents right ventricular dilatation and progression of tricuspid regurgitation in patients with tricuspid annular dilatation undergoing mitral valve repair. *J Thorac Cardiovasc Surg* 141:1431–1439.

[42] Nishimura RA, Otto CM, Bonow RO, et al. (2014) 2014 AHA/ACC Guideline for the Management of Patients With Valvular Heart Disease: Executive Summary. *Circulation* 129:2440–2492.

[43] Baumgartner H, Falk V, Bax JJ, et al. (2017) 2017 ESC/EACTS guidelines for the management of valvular heart disease. *Eur Heart J* 38:2739–2791.

[44] Dreyfus GD, Corbi PJ, Chan KMJ, Bahrami T (2005) Secondary tricuspid regurgitation or dilatation: which should be the criteria for surgical repair? *Ann Thorac Surg* 79:127–132.

[45] Chikwe J, Itagaki S, Anyanwu A, Adams DH (2015) Impact of Concomitant Tricuspid Annuloplasty on Tricuspid Regurgitation, Right Ventricular Function, and Pulmonary Artery Hypertension After Repair of Mitral Valve Prolapse. *J Am Coll Cardiol* 65:1931–1938.

[46] Kilic A, Saha-Chaudhuri P, Rankin JS, Conte JV (2013) Trends and outcomes of tricuspid valve surgery in North America: an analysis of more than 50,000 patients from the Society of Thoracic Surgeons database. *Ann Thorac Surg* 96:1546–1552; discussion 1552.

[47] Beckmann A, Meyer R, Lewandowski J, Frie M, Markewitz A, Harringer W (2018) German Heart Surgery Report 2017: The Annual Updated Registry of the German Society for Thoracic and Cardiovascular Surgery. *Thorac Cardiovasc Surg* 66:608–621.

[48] Zack CJ, Fender EA, Chandrashekar P, Reddy YNV, Bennett CE, Stulak JM, Miller VM, Nishimura RA (2017) National Trends and Outcomes in Isolated Tricuspid Valve Surgery. *J Am Coll Cardiol* 70:2953–2960.

[49] Kim Y-J, Kwon D-A, Kim H-K, et al. (2009) Determinants of surgical outcome in patients with isolated tricuspid regurgitation.

[50] De Vega N (1972) La anuloplastica selective, regulable y permanente. *Rev Esp Cardiol* 555–556.

[51] Cabrol C (1972) [Valvular annuloplasty. A new method]. *Nouv Presse Med* 1:1366.

[52] Antunes MJ, Girdwood RW (1983) Tricuspid annuloplasty: a modified technique. *Ann Thorac Surg* 35:676–678.

[53] Revuelta JM, Garcia-Rinaldi R (1989) Segmental tricuspid annuloplasty: a new technique. *J Thorac Cardiovasc Surg* 97:799–801.

[54] Onoda K, Yasuda F, Takao M, Shimono T, Tanaka K, Shimpo H, Yada I (2000) Long-term follow-up after Carpentier-Edwards ring annuloplasty for tricuspid regurgitation. *Ann Thorac Surg* 70:796–799.

[55] Tang GHL, David TE, Singh SK, Maganti MD, Armstrong S, Borger MA (2006) Tricuspid valve repair with an annuloplasty ring results in improved long-term outcomes. *Circulation* 114:I577-581.

[56] Park Y-H, Song J-M, Lee E-Y, Kim Y-J, Kang D-H, Song J-K (2008) Geometric and hemodynamic determinants of functional tricuspid regurgitation: a real-time three-dimensional echocardiography study. *Int J Cardiol* 124:160–165.

[57] Filsoufi F, Salzberg SP, Abascal V, Adams DH (2006) Surgical management of functional tricuspid regurgitation with a new remodeling annuloplasty ring. *Mt Sinai J Med* N Y 73:874–879.

[58] Navia JL, Nowicki ER, Blackstone EH, Brozzi NA, Nento DE, Atik FA, Rajeswaran J, Gillinov AM, Svensson LG, Lytle BW (2010) Surgical management of secondary tricuspid valve regurgitation: annulus, commissure, or leaflet procedure? *J Thorac Cardiovasc Surg* 139:1473-1482.e5.

[59] Fukuda S, Gillinov AM, McCarthy PM, Matsumura Y, Thomas JD, Shiota T (2007) Echocardiographic follow-up of tricuspid annuloplasty with a new three-dimensional ring in patients with functional tricuspid regurgitation. *J Am Soc Echocardiogr Off Publ Am Soc Echocardiogr* 20:1236–1242.

[60] Alfieri O, Bonis MD, Lapenna E, Agricola E, Quarti A, Maisano F (2003) The "clover technique" as a novel approach for correction of post-traumatic tricuspid regurgitation. *J Thorac Cardiovasc Surg* 126:75–79.

[61] Lapenna E, Bonis MD, Verzini A, Canna GL, Ferrara D, Calabrese MC, Taramasso M, Alfieri O (2010) The clover technique for the treatment of complex tricuspid valve insufficiency: midterm clinical and echocardiographic results in 66 patients. *Eur J Cardiothorac Surg* 37:1297–1303.

[62] Dreyfus GD, Raja SG, John Chan KM (2008) Tricuspid leaflet augmentation to address severe tethering in functional tricuspid regurgitation. *Eur J Cardio-Thorac Surg Off J Eur Assoc Cardio-Thorac Surg* 34:908–910.

[63] Solinas M, Bianchi G, Glauber M (2013) An easy and reproducible technique to address tricuspid valve regurgitation with patch augmentation. *J Card Surg* 28:638–640.

In: The Rediscovered Tricuspid Valve
Editor: Giacomo Bianchi
ISBN: 978-1-53616-098-7

Chapter 13

NOVEL TRANSCATHETER THERAPIES FOR TREATING TRICUSPID REGURGITATION

Mizuki Miura, MD, Francesco Maisano, MD, PhD, Oscar Cuevas, MD, Mara Gavazzoni, MD, Alberto Pozzoli, MD and Maurizio Taramasso*, PhD

Heart Valve Clinic, University Hospital of Zurich, Zurich, Switzerland

ABSTRACT

Tricuspid valve (TV) disease is no longer forgotten valve. High mortality and high morbidity are observed in the case of TV surgery, resulting in a lot of untreated patients in the world, but the prognosis of those patients is also extremely poor.

Transcatheter therapies for treating TR have been emerging as alternative option for patients with severe symptomatic TR and high-risk surgical condition. Although initial results from the international multicenter registry recently showed transcatheter TV therapy is feasible and safe with various techniques, clinical experience is still developing.

* Corresponding Author's E-mail: Maurizio.Taramasso@usz.ch.

Here we describe currently available technologies of transcateter TV intervention and the preliminary clinical results.

Keywords: tricuspid valve, tricuspid regurgitation, transcatheter therapy

INTRODUCTION

Tricuspid valve (TV) disease has been relatively neglected for a long time, but recently tricuspid regurgitation (TR) has attracted attention. There are about 1.6 million patients in the United State, meanwhile among them, less than 8,000 undergo TV surgery annually [1]. The prevalence of severe TR is associated with poor prognosis [2–4].

The indications of TV surgery are surgical repair of concomitant TR during left-sided valve surgery in patients with tricuspid annular dilatation or isolated TV surgery. Guidelines of TR mainly described about the former, but the main problem in daily clinical practice is the latter. 2017 ESC/EACTS guidelines described that TV surgery should be considered in patients with severe TR who are symptomatic or have progressive right ventricle (RV) dilatation/dysfunction, in the absence of severe RV dysfunction or left ventricle (LV) dysfunction and severe pulmonary vascular disease/hypertention [5], but it is difficult to assess the RV dysfunction. In addition, symptoms of right heart failure, for example leg edema, abdominal distension, hepatobiliary enzyme elevation, thrombocytopenia and so on, are more nonspecific and more confusing than symptoms of left heart failure. Futhermore the severity of TR easily changes by diuretics. Whether it applies to guidelines if TR is continuously severe or if it TR is severe even once, is not certain. Isolated TV surgery is usually performed with a very high mortality and morbidity [6–8] and do not vary across the long-term period [9]. These result in a lot of untreated patients.

Percutaneous TV therapies have been emerging as alternative option for patients with severe symptomatic TR and high-risk surgical condition [10–12]. Although initial results from the international multicenter TriValve Registry recently showed transcatheter TV therapy is feasible and safe with various techniques, clinical experience is still developing and clinical efficacy requires further investigation [13].

This review will summarize and introduce the available technologies of transcateter TV intervention and the preliminary clinical results.

SURGICAL TREATMENT

The standard surgical treatment of functional TR is tricuspid annuloplasty because the main etiology of TR is dilated tricuspid annulus. In addition, in-hospital mortality for TV replacement was significant higher than TV repair (odds ratio: 1.91, 95% CI 1.18-3.09, p=0.009) [9]. There are two methods of tricuspid annuloplasty: ring annuloplasty and suture annuloplasty. Because of good results, ring annuloplasty is more widely performed [14].

TRANSCATHETER TRICUSPID VALVE INTERVENTION

The procedures that have been developed for transcateter TV intervention are divided according to the therapeutic target; leaflet repair, annuloplasty, caval vein implantation and transcatheter tricuspid valve replacement (Figure 1).

Initial results from the international multicenter TriValve Registry recently showed transcatheter TV therapy is feasible and safe with multiple techniques [13]. Among 106 patients with severe, symptomatic TR, 68% of the cases were performed as an isolated intervention and procedural success was 62% of the cases. At 30-day follow-up, all-cause mortality was 3.7% with significant reduction of TR and symptomatic improvement.

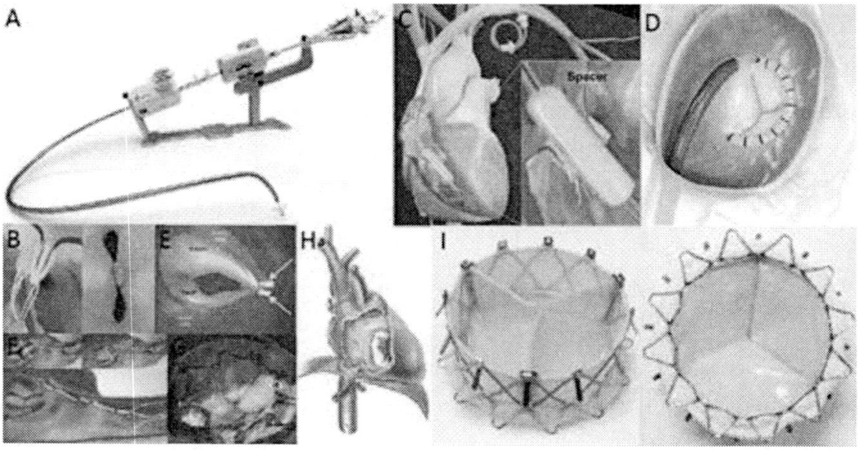

Figure 1. Transcatheter tricuspid devices. (A) MitraClip, (B) PASCAL (C) Forma, (D) Cardioband, (E) Trialign, (F) Tricinch, (G) Millipede, (H) Caval valve implantation (TricValve), (I) NaviGate.

Tricuspid Leaflet Repair

MitraClip (Abbott Vascular, Santa Clara, CA, USA) was developed as a percutaneous means to reduce MR of both degenerative and functional etiology. Now it has been successfully used for treating not only MR but also TR in selected patients [15, 16].

The procedure has been performed via transfemoal or transjugular venous approach, the former is preferred most frequently. More than 650 procedures have already been performed world wide, and 55% of the patients included in the first international registry assessing the transcatheter TR intervention underwent this therapy [13].

In contrast to the mitral valve, the use of the MitraClip system for the TR raised some specific problems due to the complexity of the TV. Therefore, intra-procedural imagings are very important (Figure 2). The use of transesophageal echocardiography (TEE) is a gold standard, but we usually combine fluoroscopy, transthoracic echocardiography (TTE) and intracardiac echocardiography (ICE).

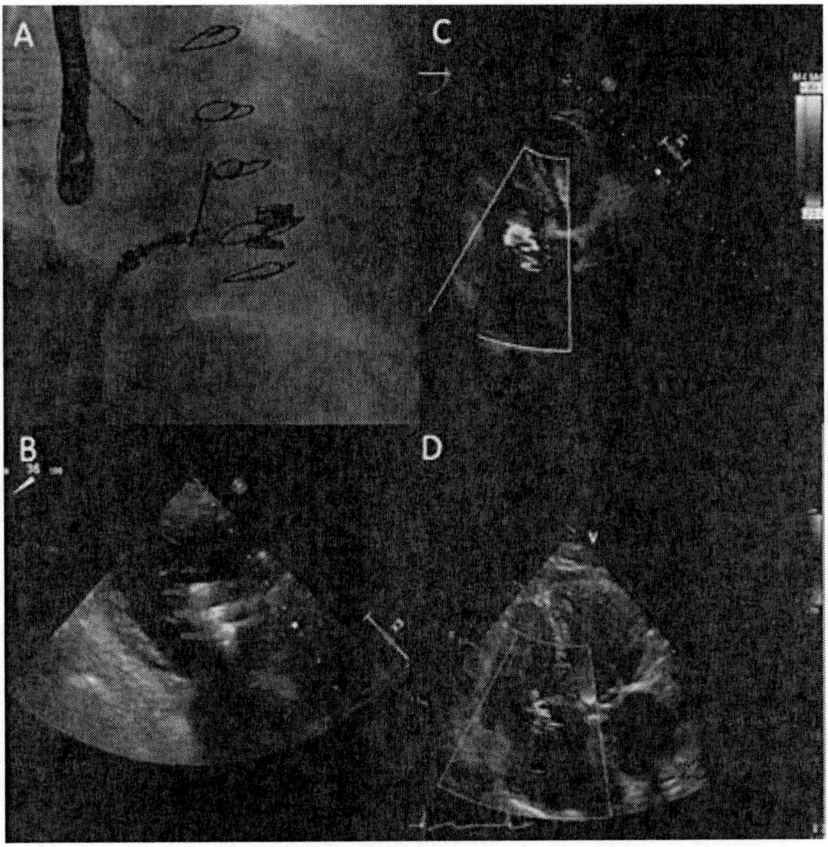

Figure 2. MitraClip for Tricuspid Regurgitation. (A) Intraprocedural Fluoroscopy. (B) Intraprocedural Transesophageal Echocardiography showing clipping the antero-septal commissure (arrow). (C) Preprocedural Transthoracic Echocardiography showing severe tricusp tricuspid regurgitation. (D) Postprocedural Transthoracic Echocardiography showing reduction of tricuspid regurgitation from severe to mild.

Fusion imagings such as the EchoNavigator (Philips) are also expected to improve introprocedural imaging technique. And the standard technique of the MitraClip system had limited steering options due to the proximity of the inferior vena cava orifice to the atrial septum as well as the short distance of the inferior vena cava orifica to the tricuspid valve coaptation line, so it is difficult to steer of the MitraClip system perpendicular to the tricuspid valve. To get rid of these limitations, the Munich technique, consisting in inserting the clip delivery system 90° counterclockwise from its typical position, is used generally [16].Therapeutic target is to reduce the effective regurgitant orifice area by closing part of the valve and reducing the defect of coaptation meanwhile regurgitation is usually central, with a large defect of coaptation. In most cases, the therapeutic goal is achieved by clipping the antero-septal commissure, which is the easiest target, and often requiring multiple grasping attempts and clips.

Nickenig et al., recently reported the 30-day outcomes in 64 consecutive severe TR patients deemed unsuitable for surgery who underwent MitraClip in a multicenter European registry. Of these, 88% of patients had functional TR and 22 patients underwent concomitant mitral repair. Procedural success was 97% and over 1 TR grade reduction was seen in 91% of patients. No life-threatening intraprocedural complications occurred, with 3 in-hospital deaths. Most patients achieved the significant reduction of TR, NYHA functional class and exercide capacity enhancement during 30-day follow-up [15].

Orban et al., reported the 6-month outcomes of 50 patients treated with MitraClip. 14 patients were treated for isolated TR and 36 patients for combained mitral regurgitation and TR. Procedural success was in 92% with a mean 1.9 clips per patient. At 6-month follow-up, a persistent reduction of at least one echocardiographic TR grade was achieved in 90% of patients and NZHA clss improved in 79% of patients. The improvements were comparable in patients undergoing isolated TR or combined MR and TR treatment. Durign follow-up, mortality was 16% and 28% of patients were hospitalized for worsening of heart failure and 4% of patients underwent TV surgery. The long-term follow-up data is expected [17].

The Edwards *PASCAL* transcatheter mitral valve repair system (Edwards Lifesciences, Irvine, CA, USA) was also developed as a percutaneous means to reduce MR of both degenerative and functional etiology. The PASCAL implant consists of a 10 mm central spacer which acts as a filter in the regurgitation orifice of the mitral valve, and is attached to the leaflets by two paddled and claps. The first-in-mad multicenter prospective observational study for mitral regurgitation showed the feasibility, safety and significant reduction of regurgitation

[18]. The first successful case for transcatheter TV repair using the PASCAL was recently reported [19].

The *FORMA* system (Edwards Lifesciences, Irvine, CA, USA) is a spacer device implanted within the tricuspid valve over a rail which is an anchored at right ventricle apex. It is designed to reduce regurgitation by occupying the regurgitant orifice area and providing a surface for the native leaflets to coapt. Introduced through a venous subclavian access, the device is locked proximally, the surplus rail is coiled and placed in a subcutaneous pocket.

Perlman et al., recently reported the 1-year clinical and echocardiographic results of the first 18 patients. Procedural success was achieved in 89%. Despite variable success in reducing echocardiographic TR grade, significant clinical improvements and reduction in right ventricular dimensions were observed at follow-up [20].

Annuloplasty Devices

The *Cardioband* system (Edwards Lifesciences, Irvine, CA, USA) is a transfemoral fully percutaneous direct annuloplasty device, which gained CE mark approval for the treatment of not only MR but also TR in April 2018 (Figure 3). It is the first commercially available transcatheter device for the TV disease. A surgical-like band is delivered into the right atrium and is implanted on the arterial side of the tricuspid annulus by means of multiple anchor elements. Final adjustment of Cardioband size by TEE and fluoroscopy under beating-heart conditions provides a reduction of the annular dimension with consequent improvement of leaflet coaptation.

The procedure has a risk of impinging right coronary artery. Preliminary results from the Cardioband Tricuspid system have been recently presented in EuroPCR 2018, Paris, France. Procedural success was achieved in 100%. 30 days-mortality was 6.7%. And Cardioband provided significant reduction in effective regurgitant orifice area (EROA) by about 50% through annular reduction. Clinically significant improvements including in functional status, quality of life (QOL) and exercise tolerability were observed at 30 days and at 6 months [21].

The *Trialign* system (Mitralign, Inc. Tewksbury, MA, USA) is designed to perform a transcatheter suture bicsupization of the TV via a transvenous jugular approach. Cinching tricuspid annulus (TA) with one or multiple pairs of pledgets enables the leaflets to get better coaptation. The procedure is carried out under general anesthesia with TEE guidance.US multicenter prospective registry study (SCOUT) recently showed the feasibility and the safety of the device during 30 days [22]. Fifteen patients with New York Heart Association (NYHA) functional class II and moderate or greater functional TR were enrolled. All patients underwent successful device implantation without death and any major adverse events. Technical success rate at 30 days was 80% (three single pledget annular detachments). Significant reduction of dilated tricuspid annulus area and effective regurgitant orifice area, as well as improvement in left ventricular stroke volume and QOL, was also observed.

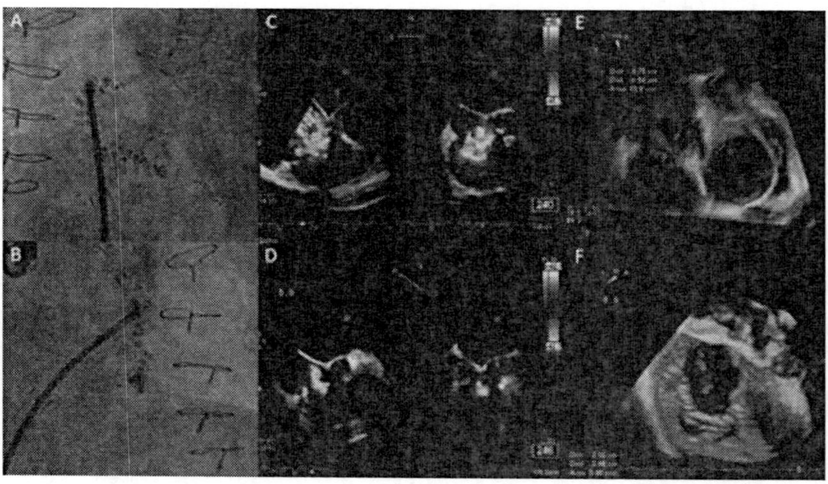

Figure 3. Cardioband for Tricuspid Regurgitation. (A) (B) Intraprocedural Fluoroscopy. (C) Preprocedural Transesophageal Echocardiography showing severe tricuspid regurgitation. (D) Postprocedural Transesophageal Echocardiography showing reduction of tricuspid r regurgitation from severe to mild after cinching. (E) Preprocedural Transesophageal Echocardiography showing expansion of tricuspid annulus. (F) Postprocedural Transesophageal Echocardiography showing decreasing the tricuspid annulus area from 15.8 cm^2 to 5.86 cm^2 after cinching.

The *TriCinch* (4 Tech Cardio, Galway, Ireland) is a percutaneous device designed to cinch dilated tricuspid annulus via transfemoral venous approach. An anchor element is implanted, usually close to anteroposterior commissure. By tensioning the anchor, annular plication is performed to reduce the tricuspid annulus area and gain better coaptation of the leaflets. Finally, a self-expandable nitinol stent, which is connected to the anchor element, is implanted in inferior vena cava. Optimal tension is maintained by the stent. The procedure is performed by using TEE and/or intracardiac echocardiography (ICE). The prospective, single arm multicenter study (PREVENT TriCinch™ European FIH Trial) is currently reported in LondonValves 2017, London, UK [23]. Among 24 patients, device success was 81% and no patients died during 30 days. Late anchor detachment was observed in 23%. This trial demonstrated acute safety and efficacy with no major adverse events, ability to reduce TR, and patient's QOL.

The *Millipede* (Millipede, LLC, Ann Arbor, MI, USA) is a direct annuloplasty device which is inserted and fixed at artrial part of the annulus surgically or by transcatheter, to restore its shape and diameter. This device mimics surgical annuloplasty and can be used for the treatment of both MR and TR. 2 cases were implanted in both mitral and tricuspid valve. Both patients experienced the reduction in tricuspid annulus diameter of 42% to 45% with no post-procedural residual TR [24].

Caval Vein Implantation

Caval vein implantation (CAVI) is an alternative concept of percutaneous treatment of TV. Caval valve prosthesis are implanted via transvenous approach in inferior vena cava (IVC) or in combination with a superior vena cava (SVC) valve (BiCAVI) to reduce venous backflow and right heart strain, thus result in preventing damage to liver and other organs. The self-expandable TricValve (P&F, Vienna, Austria), the balloon-expandable valve (SAPIEN XT/3, Edwards Lifesciences, Irvine, CA, USA), and other devices (Directflow, Direct Flow Medical, Santa Rosa, CA, USA) have been used for CAVI. TricValve consists of two self-expandable biological valves. It has been specifically developed for the low-pressure venous, and is implanted percutaneously into IVC and SVC without disturbing the native tricuspid valve.

Among 25 patients treated in multicenter observational First-in-Man study of CAVI, the device was successfully implanted in 96% cases [25]. In 2 cases (8%), the prosthetic valves were surgically removed because of the device migration within 30 days. CAVI resulted in complete reduction or reserve caval flow in all patients and symptoms improved in 84.2% by 1 or more NYHA class. Thirty-day mortality was 12% and 12-month mortality was 63%. Mean follow-up time after CAVI was 316±453 days (14-1540 days), and no degenerative prosthetic valves were seen.

Transcatheter Tricuspid Valve Replacement

The *NaviGate* bioprosthesis (NaviGate Cardiac Structures, Inc, Laguna Hills, CA, USA) is a novel self-expandable valve designed to treat functional tricuspid regurgitation. It is the only device that has been used to perform transcatheter tricuspid valve implantation. The procedure is usually performed via transatrial or transjugular access (Figure 4).

Navia JL et al., demonstrated the feasibility of transcatheter tricuspid valve implantation using the NaviGate valved-stent in a long-term swine model [26]. Excellent hemodynamic and valve performance were observed without any major complications. First-in-human successful implantation of the NaviGate valved-stent in 2 cases was recently reported [27]. One was implanted via transatrial approach with mild to moderate paravalvular TR, and the other was implanted via transjugular approach with mild mild TR. The short-term results suggest that NaviGate is safe and feasible using transatrial or transjugular approaches.

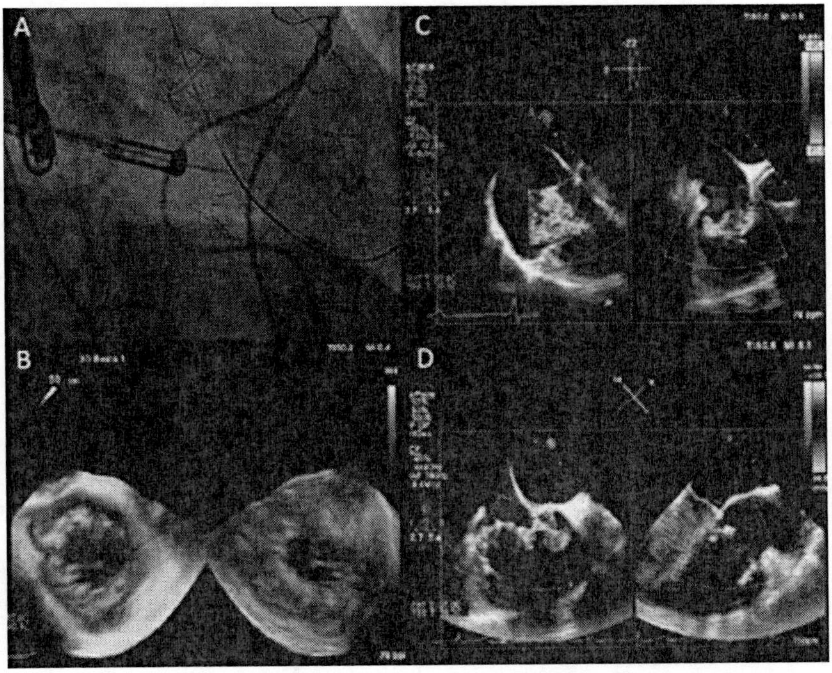

Figure 4. NaviGate for Tricuspid Regurgitation. (A) Intraprocedural Fluoroscopy. (B) Transesophageal Echocardiography after Implantation. (C) Preprocedural Transesophageal Echocardiography showing severe tricuspid regurgitation. (D) Postprocedural Transesophageal Echocardiography showing reduction of tricuspid regurgitation from severe to trivial.

Conclusion

Recently, TV disease is occupying the spotlight and transcatheter TV therapy is rapidly developing. Patients who are treated with transcatheter therapy are mostly high-risk functional severe TR patients with no severely impaired RV function. Initial results suggest that transcatheter TV therapy is feasible and safe with different techniques, but clinical efficacy is still to be proven. Further investigation is needed to assess indication, patient selection, anatomical eligibility, long-term outcome and optimal procedural timing.

REFERENCES

[1] Stuge O, Liddicoat J (2006) Emerging opportunities for cardiac surgeons within structural heart disease. *J. Thorac. Cardiovasc. Surg.* 132:1258–1261.

[2] Nath J, Foster E, Heidenreich PA (2004) Impact of Tricuspid Regurgitation on Long-Term Survival. *J. Am. Coll. Cardiol.* 43:405–409.

[3] Agricola E, Stella S, Gullace M, Ingallina G, D'Amato R, Slavich M, Oppizzi M, Ancona MB, Margonato A (2012) Impact of functional tricuspid regurgitation on heart failure and death in patients with functional mitral regurgitation and left ventricular dysfunction. *Eur. J. Heart Fail.* 14:902–908.

[4] Topilsky Y, Nkomo VT, Vatury O, et al. (2014) Clinical Outcome of Isolated Tricuspid Regurgitation. *JACC Cardiovasc. Imaging.* 7:1185–1194.

[5] Baumgartner H, Falk V, Bax JJ, et al. (2017) 2017 ESC/EACTS guidelines for the management of valvular heart disease. *Eur. Heart J.* 38:2739–2791.

[6] Chang B-C, Lim S-H, Yi G, Hong YS, Lee S, Yoo K-J, Kang MS, Cho BK (2006) Long-term clinical results of tricuspid valve replacement. *Ann. Thorac. Surg.* 81:1317–1324.

[7] Kaplan M, Kut MS, Demirtas MM, Cimen S, Ozler A (2002) Prosthetic replacement of tricuspid valve: bioprosthetic or mechanical. *Ann. Thorac. Surg.* 73:467–473.

[8] Songur CM, Simsek E, Ozen A, Kocabeyoglu S, Donmez TA (2014) Long term results comparing mechanical and biological prostheses in the tricuspid valve position: which valve types are better--mechanical or biological prostheses? *Heart Lung Circ.* 23:1175–1178.

[9] Zack CJ, Fender EA, Chandrashekar P, Reddy YNV, Bennett CE, Stulak JM, Miller VM, Nishimura RA (2017) National Trends and Outcomes in Isolated Tricuspid Valve Surgery. *J. Am. Coll. Cardiol.* 70:2953–2960.

[10] Rodés-Cabau J, Taramasso M, O'Gara PT (2016) Diagnosis and treatment of tricuspid valve disease: current and future perspectives. *The Lancet* 388:2431–2442.

[11] Taramasso M, Pozzoli A, Guidotti A, Nietlispach F, Inderbitzin DT, Benussi S, Alfieri O, Maisano F (2017) Percutaneous tricuspid valve therapies: the new frontier. *Eur. Heart J.* 38:639–647.

[12] Taramasso M, Maisano F (2017) Novel Technologies for percutaneous treatment of tricuspid valve regurgitation. *Eur. Heart J.* 38:2707–2710.

[13] Taramasso M, Hahn RT, Alessandrini H, et al. (2017) The International Multicenter TriValve Registry: Which Patients Are Undergoing Transcatheter Tricuspid Repair? *JACC Cardiovasc. Interv.* 10:1982–1990.

[14] Onoda K, Yasuda F, Takao M, Shimono T, Tanaka K, Shimpo H, Yada I (2000) Long-term follow-up after Carpentier-Edwards ring annuloplasty for tricuspid regurgitation. *Ann. Thorac. Surg.* 70:796–799.

[15] Nickenig G, Kowalski M, Hausleiter J, et al. (2017) Transcatheter Treatment of Severe Tricuspid Regurgitation With the Edge-to-Edge MitraClip Technique. *Circulation* 135:1802–1814.

[16] Braun D, Orban M, Nabauer M, et al. (2017) Transcatheter Treatment of Severe Tricuspid Regurgitation Using the Edge-to-Edge Repair Technique in the Presence and Absence of Pacemaker Leads. *JACC Cardiovasc. Interv.* 10:2014–2016.

[17] Orban M, Besler C, Braun D, et al. (2018) Six-month outcome after transcatheter edge-to-edge repair of severe tricuspid regurgitation in patients with heart failure. *Eur. J. Heart Fail.* 20:1055–1062.

[18] Praz F, Spargias K, Chrissoheris M, et al. (2017) Compassionate use of the PASCAL transcatheter mitral valve repair system for patients with severe mitral regurgitation: a multicentre, prospective, observational, first-in-man study. *Lancet Lond. Engl.* 390:773–780.

[19] Fam NP, Ho EC, Zahrani M, Samargandy S, Connelly KA (2018) Transcatheter Tricuspid Valve Repair With the PASCAL System. *JACC Cardiovasc. Interv.* 11:407–408.

[20] Perlman G, Praz F, Puri R, et al. (2017) Transcatheter Tricuspid Valve Repair with a New Transcatheter Coaptation System for the Treatment of Severe Tricuspid Regurgitation: 1-Year Clinical and Echocardiographic Results. *JACC Cardiovasc. Interv.* 10:1994–2003.

[21] Von Bardeleben RS (2018) *How Cardioband Tricuspid System can benefit my patients.*

[22] Hahn RT, Meduri CU, Davidson CJ, et al. (2017) Early Feasibility Study of a Transcatheter Tricuspid Valve Annuloplasty: SCOUT Trial 30-Day Results. *J. Am. Coll. Cardiol.* 69:1795–1806.

[23] Denti P (2017) *4Tech-Clinical Outcomes and Current Challenges.*

[24] Rogers JH (2017) *Millipede for TR: Technique and Outcomes.*

[25] Lauten A, Figulla HR, Unbehaun A, et al. (2018) Interventional Treatment of Severe Tricuspid Regurgitation: Early Clinical Experience in a Multicenter, Observational, First-in-Man Study. *Circ. Cardiovasc. Interv.* 11:e006061.

[26] Navia JL, Kapadia S, Elgharably H, Maluenda G, Bartuś K, Baeza C, Nair RK, Rodés-Cabau J, Beghi C, Quijano RC (2018) Transcatheter Tricuspid Valve Implantation of NaviGate Bioprosthesis in a Preclinical Model. *JACC Basic Transl. Sci.* 3:67–79.

[27] Navia JL, Kapadia S, Elgharably H, et al. (2017) First-in-Human Implantations of the NaviGate Bioprosthesis in a Severely Dilated Tricuspid Annulus and in a Failed Tricuspid Annuloplasty Ring. *Circ. Cardiovasc. Interv.* doi: 10.1161/circinterventions.117.0058 40.

About the Editor

Giacomo Bianchi MD, PhD

Consultant Cardiac Surgeon at Ospedale del Cuore – Fondazione Toscana "G. Monasterio", Massa, Italy

Scuola Superiore Sant'Anna, Pisa, Italy

Giacomo Bianchi is Consultant Cardiac Surgeon at the Cardiothoracic Department of the Ospedale del Cuore "G. Pasquinucci" – Fondazione Toscana G. Monasterio in Massa.

Dr. Bianchi worked in the United States for about (2009-2010) 12 months at the "Artificial Organs Lab" of the University of Maryland, Baltimore. There he acquired the techniques of cell culture and molecular analysis with cytofluorimeter, PCR and western blotting; in this place he performed implants of ventricular assist devices (Jarvick child size) and ECMO.

In December 2013 Dr. Bianchi obtained the Diploma di Perfezionamento (Doctorate of Philosophy, PhD) in the Curriculum of "Molecular Medicine and Genomic Physiology" at the Scuola Superiore Sant'Anna in Pisa, defending the experimental thesis of "Gene therapy in a mouse model of aneurysm of the ascending thoracic aorta". During this training period he perfected the techniques of western blotting, cell culture and production of lentiviral vectors.

For the entire duration of his doctorate, he also continued to work as a cardiac surgeon at the Ospedale del Cuore.

Dr. Bianchi's current interests are focused on minimally invasive surgical techniques of aortic (minitoracotomy, ministernotomy) and mitral ± tricuspid (minitoracotomy) valve repair and replacement; the latter aspect has recently been implemented through the adoption of an endoscopic approach (periareolar video assisted mini-thoracotomy).

In addition, thanks to the experience borrowed in the United States, Dr. Bianchi is interested in the surgical treatment of heart failure (end-stage revascularization, mitral and tricuspid surgery, cardiac transplantation, ventricular assist devices).

Other interests: statistics, R, reproducible research; python for data analysis; machine learning

INDEX

C

D

E

F

G

H

I

J

K

L

M

N

O

P

Q

R

U

V

W

Related Nova Publications

A Closer Look at Cardiovascular Diseases and Risk Factors

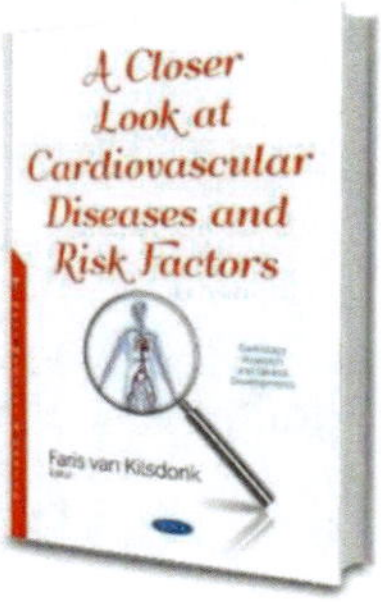

Editor: Faris van Kilsdonk

Series: Cardiology Research and Clinical Developments

Book Description: In recent decades, obesity levels have increased worldwide, thus also increasing the prevalence of morbid obesity. This type of obesity is associated with a large number of comorbidities that increase the mortality risk of the patients who suffer it.

Softcover ISBN: 978-1-53613-939-6
Retail Price: $95

Myocardial Perfusion Imaging (MPI): Performance, Potential Risks and Outcomes

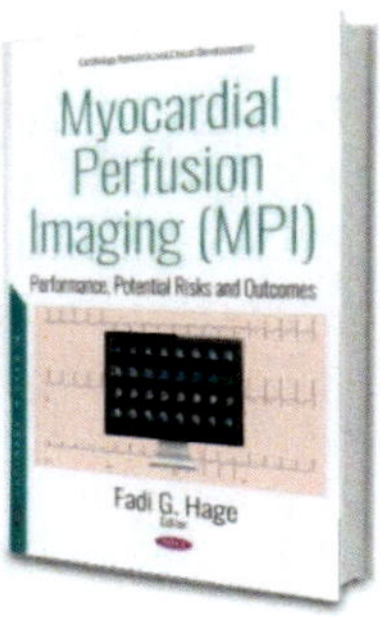

Editor: Fadi Gabriel Hage, M.D.

Series: Cardiology Research and Clinical Developments

Book Description: Myocardial perfusion imaging (MPI) is the most commonly used non-invasive stress imaging test for the diagnosis and risk stratification of coronary artery disease. Although MPI has been around for decades, recent advances have made possible fundamental changes in the performance of this test.

Hardcover ISBN: 978-1-53613-476-6
Retail Price: $310